Matron at Last

Also by Evelyn Prentis

A Nurse in Time
A Nurse in Action
A Nurse and Mother

Matron at Last

The True Story of a Nurse Turned Matron

EVELYN PRENTIS

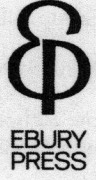

EBURY
PRESS

1 3 5 7 9 10 8 6 4 2

Published in 2012 by Ebury Press, an imprint of Ebury Publishing
A Random House Group company
First published in Great Britain by
Hutchinson & Co (Publishers) Ltd in 1981

The Random House Group Limited Reg. No. 954009

Addresses for companies within the Random House Group can be
found at www.randomhouse.co.uk

A CIP catalogue record for this book is available from the British Library

The Random House Group Limited supports The Forest Stewardship
Council (FSC®), the leading international forest certification
organisation. Our books carrying the FSC label are printed on FSC®
certified paper. FSC is the only forest certification scheme endorsed
by the leading environmental organisations, including Greenpeace.
Our paper procurement policy can be found at
www.randomhouse.co.uk/environment

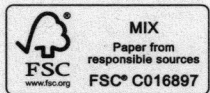

Printed and bound by CPI Group (UK) Ltd, Croydon, CR0 4YY

ISBN 9780091941390

To buy books by your favourite authors and register for offers visit
www.randomhouse.co.uk

For Toby, Ben and Wimpy

Part One

Part One

Chapter One

WHEN THE DAY came for me to take off my uniform for the last time and bring to an end thirty years of being a hospital nurse (less the few I spent at home steering the children through teething troubles, infant school traumas and all the other little difficulties, which growing up to be round about seven had caused), it was as if I was saying farewell to an old friend. But I bore up bravely. I wiped away a tear, threw a last look over my shoulder at the nurses who were waving to me from the locker room door, and rode off home. It was the end of a chapter and I wasn't sure how the next one would begin.

Though I had never been able to boast that I was a born nurse, I had been a nurse long enough to know that I could never have been anything else once I got over the shock of a stern and chilly Matron and some very niggly ward sisters. Scrubbing walls, scouring bedpans or picking nits out of heads wasn't the most glamorous start to a career, but being a probationer in the thirties meant that I had to do the scrubbing, scouring and nit-picking with as good a grace as possible until I was senior enough to be more selective in what I did.

Not being a born nurse made everything doubly difficult in the days when having a vocation that shone as brightly as Miss Nightingale's lamp was the only justification for a girl to sew name tapes on her under-wear, pack a portmanteau and go off to be a nurse. A starting salary of less than twenty pounds a year was never intended as bait to catch the mercenary. Without the vocation there had to be some tremendous compulsion for taking such a drastic step. Or a very determined mother.

My mother had always yearned to be a nurse herself, and had followed the doctor for years. 'Following the doctor' meant rushing off at a moment's notice when an extra pair of hands was needed to help with a difficult confinement; or throwing a toothbrush and a nightdress into a glad-stone bag to be ready and waiting when the message was brought that her next lying-in patient was having contractions. My mother didn't call them contrac-tions. She called them labour pains, which was as good a name as any for the thrashing agony that too often spoilt the fun of having a baby before ways were thought of to make it easier for those who wanted it made easier.

But in spite of her longings to be a nurse my mother never had the opportunity to do her training. She had to be satisfied with following the doctor, and probably saw in me the realizations of her own thwarted ambitions. Though whether the carefully posed, oh-so-natural picture of me in uniform that she kept on her sideboard satisfied her yearnings I never knew. She didn't waste time indulging in sentimental disclosures and had little patience with those who did.

For a year or two after my father died she had lived alone, proudly refusing to listen when we begged her to uproot herself and move from the depths of Lincolnshire to the outskirts of London to be with her family. I waited until she was too frail to argue, then I resigned from the hospital and went and fetched her. In less time than it took to bring her from her house to ours she had forgotten most of the faces and places she had left behind.

Having her to live with us was very much nicer than we had thought it would be. Remembering the spirited woman she once was, I had expected some of her old fieriness still to be there, flaring up often and making us all shrink back while the heat was on. But there was no fire left in her. Instead of disrupting the house with her difficult little ways as she would once have done, she endowed it with a special sort of warmth that more than rewarded us for turning the spare room into a granny room and later rearranging the sitting-room furniture so that she didn't have to climb the stairs to go to bed.

The very old are often to be pitied. Senility can be a cruelly distressing thing; a lingering illness, even if born with patience, can be the sad end of a long and useful life. Senile my mother was, but not cruelly so. She lived in a past that almost totally blotted out the present and saw in the unfamiliar surroundings of her strange new home the familiar scenes of her girlhood days. She greeted those she had never set eyes on before with the delight of one who has suddenly been reunited with an old and valued friend and she put the clock back for them as she did for herself.

'My, but you've grown since I saw you last,' she exclaimed in wonder to the butcher's boy, who only delivered at weekends and Christmas to eke out his old age pension.

'And what a fine lad you are,' she said to the baker's roundsman, who was already trying to make up his mind whether to take a cheque or insist on a marble clock as a retirement gift.

'Fancy you being a doctor,' she cried to the strapping young man who dropped in daily to see how she was, and twice a day when her heart started failing. 'The spit of your father as well, though if I remember rightly your mother was never too sure about him. A rum lot she turned out to be and no mistake.'

Each of them was unfailingly kind and listened patiently while she told them of the pranks their parents got up to when she and they were at school together. They occasionally added a spicy detail themselves to the stories she told them, blackening their alleged father's character to such a degree that she flushed uncomfortably at having caused the skeleton in their cupboard to rattle its bones. When they had gone she would fall into a reverie of recollection, talking softly to the invisibles in the room and chuckling at the things they said to her. It was a joy having my mother living with us. We only wished she could have stayed longer.

When she died, quite peacefully one Sunday, we moved her bed out of the sitting room, put the furniture back in its proper place and life went on as if she had never been there – but with one important difference. I was no longer a part-time nurse, fitting in being a wife and mother between the spells of duty at the hospital. I was a full-time housewife with nothing to do but sweep and scrub, dust and polish, wash and cook, with a bit of gardening to fill the idle hours.

The feeling of freedom was fine at first. There was no turning out on my rackety old bicycle to go to work, no frail mother needing constant care, and now, of course, no small children clamouring for attention just when I was settling down to have a quiet read.

The children were children no longer. There was already the glint of engagement rings and the whispering of wedding plans behind closed doors, accompanied by the wailing of the Beatles and the impassioned throb of Elvis. Soon I would be a mother-in-law and a prop for comedians to use when they needed material for their music-hall jokes.

I wasn't dismayed by the prospect. I had never dreaded the day when I would turn up at church looking every inch the bride's mother, petalled hat and matching bag and shoes. I knew I would be able to force a smile while I was throwing confetti even if I had wept buckets during the service. I also rather fancied myself as a grandma should the day ever come. The name had an old-fashioned ring which would suit me fine. I could hardly wait.

When the joys of not having to go to work began to pall, I started looking for things to do that would fill the idle hours when I wasn't weeding the garden. I had never been held captive by the repetitive round of housework. Fingerprints on paintwork failed to throw me into a state of manic depression and fluff under the beds didn't worry me as long as it stayed where I couldn't see it. I dusted a room or swept a floor when driven by conscience rather than because it was the appointed time for sweeping and dusting. I was addicted to neither.

Nor was I an enthusiastic knitter. The sight of a ball of wool steadily shrinking until it became a garment had never inspired me with the urge to create. I had painstakingly purled and plained while the children were too young to worry about the misfits they were made to wear, but as they got older and started asking awkward questions about dropped stitches I gave up knitting and went out and bought their woollies instead.

I was as unskilled at sewing as I was at knitting. This I blamed on my mother. I can never remember her putting a stitch into anything in time to save nine. She had postponed doing the family mending for as long as possible, forever sometimes, declaring that the very sight of a sewing needle was enough to make her quarrel with her own shadow. It was certainly enough to make her quarrel with anybody who went near her while she was doing a running repair. She sat stabbing the needle in and out of whatever she was mending with the ferocity of one wielding a lethal weapon. It was always best to keep out of her way when there was a sock needing darning.

I didn't go to such extremes but neither did I leap for the sewing box at the first report of a button becoming detached from a shirt or a suspender falling off a girdle. I allowed a decent time to elapse before attaching button to shirt or suspender to girdle and even then there was no guarantee that they would stay attached.

Once, after a friend had hinted that it was only idiots like me that couldn't sew, I enrolled at an evening class determined to learn. It wasn't as easy as falling off a log as my friend had promised. I and several other novices were led step by step through the intricacies of making a skirt. After six weeks of hard labour I held the still unfinished garment at arm's length and caught the sewing teacher's eye.

'What does it look like?' I asked, and waited for praise.

'It looks exactly like a bell tent, dear,' she said. I never went back to the sewing class. I left the bell tent behind to be cut up into several dusters and forfeited the rest of the enrolment fee.

I had just started to do the rounds of the voluntary

services to discover where my few poor talents could be put to their best use when things happened that affected me more deeply than anything had affected me before. The break-up of a marriage can never be less than painful and the break-up of mine gave everybody concerned their share of pain. It went the way of most broken marriages: first the bitter recriminations, then a slow acceptance of the inevitable, a reluctant admission that maybe, and only maybe mind you, whatever blame there was could be evenly apportioned between both sides, and afterwards a long, long period of adjustment to a different way of life. Rehabilitation was a slow process.

When the recriminations had lost some of their bitterness and the period of adjustment was getting under way, I started looking for things to do that would not only fill the idle hours but would fatten my purse. It had got much thinner while I was adjusting. I racked my brains thinking up ways of earning an honest penny. I knew no way of earning a dishonest one or I might have tried my luck at that. Desperation leads us into temptation quicker than the apple in Eden.

All I could think of while I was racking my brains was to go back to being a full-time nurse at the hospital where I had worked part-time before my mother needed looking after. But the more I thought about it, the less attractive the solution seemed. I had spent a great many years as a resident nurse. I knew only too well the restrictions I would be up against if I went to live in a nurses' home. I was past the age to want such restrictions. Though many of them had been lifted over the years, and there was now no ten o'clock curfew to have nurses scrambling into their bedroom window as I had so often scrambled into mine, and no home sister prowling the corridors ready to pounce on sinners, there were other drawbacks to being resident. If I was ever to be a grandma and play my proper part in the role there would need to be somewhere for visiting grandchildren to come and stay. However many restrictions had been lifted and however lenient the home sisters might have become, I couldn't envisage one of them throwing open the doors of the nurses' home to admit the patter of tiny feet, especially if the feet were encased in wellies and the wellies happened to be encrusted with mud. The domestics would have something to say about that as well.

Even if the home sister and the domestics could bring themselves to turn a blind eye, there would still be the night nurses to contend with. Night nurses are notoriously light sleepers. A pin has only to be dropped and they are awake, reaching for a dressing gown and storming onto the corridor to kill whoever dropped it. I could imagine them going en masse to the matron complaining that they hadn't had a wink of sleep all day what with the thundering of feet up and down the corridor and the prattle of voices outside their doors. I was determined that my grandchildren, should I ever have any, would be able to visit their grandma without encountering ogres and dragons at every step they took.

After I had finally given up the idea of becoming a full-time resident nurse I started considering the possibilities of becoming a full-time non-resident nurse. There were snags to this as well, the greatest being that to be non-resident there had to be some place for me to reside. The time was rapidly approaching when the roof over my head would have to be replaced with something that cost less to maintain in its pristine condition. This, and the slender purse, gave me headaches that aspirin failed to cure.

It had just begun to seem as if I would have to settle for the bedsitter in a nurses' home with all its drawbacks, when a Messenger of Heaven appeared before me one morning when I was doing my shopping in the High Street. Her wings and halo were so effectively hidden that I didn't recognise her as a

Heavenly Messenger. She looked exactly like one of the kind assistant nurses I had worked with when I was a part-timer at the fever hospital on the other side of the town.

We stopped, stared, then put down our shopping baskets in the middle of the pavement to the annoyance of the passers-by and prepared ourselves for a cosy session of hospital gossip. I felt a surge of excitement at the prospect. I hadn't realized until that moment how much I had missed the backbiting, the interesting bits of scandal and the friendly exchanges of domestic tragedies which part-time married nurses exult or gloom over while they are having a coffee-break or eating their meal allowance. I waited eagerly to be brought up to date with news of a wrong injection that had been given, narrowly avoiding a death-by-misadventure verdict; of a nurse who had run off with somebody else's husband or whose husband had run off with somebody else's wife. The assistant nurse spoke first.

'Hello,' she said.

'Hello,' I returned. It wasn't a promising start to an encounter that was to solve my most pressing problems.

We stood for a moment saying a few kind words about those we had a mutual liking for and denouncing the less favoured ones. When I inquired about the current staffing situation I was told that it was as it had always been, part-timers never there and the full-timers having to do all the work, plus an epidemic of something or other that was filling the cubicles. I kept discreetly silent. I had been a part-timer for ten years and knew how frustrating it was for the full-timers when a mother rang in to say she wouldn't be on duty until her children had got over the measles. It was even more frustrating when more than one mother rang on the same day.

The assistant nurse and I were still blocking the pavement when she started doing what she had been sent to do by whichever guardian angel was watching over me at that particular time.

'Where are you working now?' she asked in her flat Lincolnshire accent. Like me she had left her natural habitat to seek her fortune as a nurse on the outskirts of London, and like me she hadn't found a fortune. She was still working at the fever hospital when she should have been resting her arches.

When I told her that I wasn't working anywhere, and explained why, she made such sympathetic noises that I surprised us both by bursting into tears. We picked up our shopping baskets and hurried across the road to a small cafe. There, over a cup of tea and a well-burnt currant bun, I unburdened myself to the willing listener. I let my hair down, had a good cry and after I had blown my nose on the paper serviette that came with the bun felt almost like a new woman.

The willing listener gave me her dry serviette and ordered the same again for both of us.

'So what are you going to do about it?' she mumbled, taking a burnt currant out of her mouth and placing it on the side of her plate.

'I don't know,' I said, gulping back a sob. I had cried quite enough for one day. More than I had cried for years.

'How about coming back to the fever hospital? We could do with extra staff and you could live either in or out.' She picked another burnt currant out of her bun.

I explained about not wanting to live in, and about not having anywhere to live if I lived out. It all sounded so terribly dreary that I had to gulp even harder to stop the sob from escaping. The nurse looked thoughtfully down at the grimy table cloth. When she looked up she showed no sign that she was going to say something that would make such an impact on my life.

'One of our patients told me that they are looking for a new matron at the place for old ladies down the bottom end of the town,' she said.

'What do you know about it?' I asked her, trying not to get too excited about something that might never happen. We drank a third cup of tea while she told me all she knew. It wasn't much, but there was enough to set the church bells pealing through the town. I learned later that they were pealing for a bride who had just walked down the aisle with her brand new husband but I didn't think she would have grudged me a share in her happiness.

Apparently there was a house that went with the job; not a mansion but big enough for visiting grand-children to stay as long as they wanted, and a garden where they could get their wellies dirty without anybody minding. It sounded just the sort of paradise I had dreamed of but had never hoped to find. I thanked my kind friend for the tea and buns, which she had insisted on paying for, then we went our separate ways, she to the hospital for the afternoon shift and I back home to start writing letters that would eventually lead to me being the matron of the place for elderly ladies.

Chapter Two

IN THE TIME that elapsed between writing the first of many letters and the time I went for the first of many interviews, I was beset by the hopes and fears of every applicant for a new job. I tossed and turned at night, had nightmares during the day and dreamed dreams that didn't come true.

I thought of the homes for the elderly that were starting to spring up everywhere, red bricked and modern, chintzed and cretonned, and plentifully supplied with the most up-to-date equipment specially designed with the elderly in mind, and all heavily subsidized by public funds.

I pictured myself as the matron of just such a place, floating about and being gracious, and running my lily white hands along ledges and shelves in search of dust as the matrons of old had done. I made up kind little speeches to deliver when I was doing the rounds. I planned the exact words I would use when I was inquiring solicitously after the residents' health and the state of their bowels. Because I was a nurse I knew how important it was to inquire about bowels. To have been or not to have been was the question that had to be answered honestly at the close of every day. Not to have been could cause a lot of distress unless immediate steps were taken to restore regularity.

It required only one interview to establish how far from reality the dreams were. I quickly discovered that the place at the bottom end of the town wasn't one of the glossy modern homes, fully equipped and heavily subsidized. It was in fact a rather shabby collection of Victorian flatlets, supported by a charitable body and occupied by elderly ladies of reduced circumstances. There wasn't a single piece of modern equipment throughout the entire building.

Neither would I be the sort of matron I had envisaged. Instead of floating about and being gracious I would be kept busy answering emergency bells, arranging for new washers to be put on dripping taps, seeing that the chimneys were swept regularly and that the coal was delivered on the day it was due. There would be many other things to ensure that my hands were never lily white. I was a little upset about this. Being a matron should, I thought, have offered more scope for gracious living.

There was one other thing that troubled me ever so slightly about being employed outside the Health Service. From the time that I first started nursing I had worked under the efficient if impersonal protection of a municipal hospital. The money they paid me was never enough, but at least it was handed out regularly by one of the junior clerks out of the finance office who kept us queuing for a long time outside a little window before he condescended to hand us our pay packets. Short of a major disaster, each of us could be absolutely certain of being meagrely paid for our services once a month if we worked full time, or once a week if we were part-timers paid on an hourly basis. It had never occurred to us to wonder whether there would be enough money to go round. We took the envelope with barely a thank you.

But in the new job which I was so anxious to get I would be dependent on private enterprise for my daily bread instead of being a name and number on the public sector's expense account. There were times when I was haunted by the fear that during periods of high inflation rates or low investment returns the charitable body would forget to pay me, or would run out of funds, or would need my salary to give to the rich-turned-poor who came knocking at their door with begging bowls. I had visions of the day when I would be a beggar myself. Luckily the visions were as groundless as the fears.

It was on a balmy summer morning when I first went to look at the place where I would shortly be working. It wasn't easy to find. Though I had lived near the town since the beginning of the war when I went to be a staff nurse at the sanatorium, there were still parts of it I wasn't familiar with, and streets I had never heard of.

The street where I had been told to alight from the bus was so thick with traffic that getting from one side to the other was perilous. Rows of terraced houses were separated by a derelict Wesleyan chapel, one or two self-conscious semis, and a small wooden cabin with a board outside telling anybody who was interested that ice cream could be bought there. There were other signs saying that cigarettes could be bought there. Later I was to discover that almost everything that might be needed in a hurry could be bought from the small wooden cabin.

At the other end of the street from where the bus had dropped me a river ran under a bridge. There were swans on the river. There were also rats. I stood for a moment watching the swans floating up stream and the rats swimming from hole to hole in the muddy margins where nettles and water weeds grew. Then I walked back down the street still looking for the place where the elderly ladies lived.

'There's nowhere of that name round here,' said the first man I asked, vigorously shaking his head. 'Leastways if there is I've never heard of it and I've lived here the best part of my life. Sorry I can't help you.'

I thanked him for not being able to help me and stopped another man who looked as if he also had lived there for the best part of his life, which could even have been longer than the first man. He took his pipe out of his mouth, gazed vaguely up and down the road, looked sorrowfully at me and shook his head. 'No,' he said, 'I think you must have got the wrong road or summat. Mebbe the place you're looking for is further up and over the bridge.'

It wasn't. The man in the cabin told me that it was at the end of the cul-de-sac between the derelict Wesleyan chapel and one of the rows of terraced houses. I wondered why neither of the others had known. I had to wait awhile before I found the answer to that.

At the end of the cul-de-sac and opposite a wide macadamed forecourt stood a two-storeyed white-washed building, crescent shaped and gabled. A dozen or more latticed windows on the upper floor caught and threw back beams from the morning sun. Between the windows on the ground floor, heavy doors which led to I knew not where were all firmly shut, and from tall Victorian chimneys puffs of smoke gently polluted the summer air.

Along the front of the building ran a verandah bright with flowers that spilled out of hanging baskets; a porch in the middle of the verandah had splashes of scarlet geraniums on its white painted walls. From where I stood I could smell the roses that dropped a confetti of petals on the green lawns, but except for a sleeping cat and a wide variety of bird life there wasn't a soul in sight.

The cat was several shades of ginger. It was spread out under the shade of two trees and looked so vulnerable, innocently sleeping and dreaming of mice, that I could never have guessed that the day would come when I would be wishing it was anywhere but there. The ginger cat became a thorn in my flesh that was to influence my prayers and have me beseeching the Lord in His mercy to do something about it. I realized later that it wasn't dreaming of mice when it slept, it was dreaming up ways of making my life a misery and putting bad thoughts into my heart and wicked words into my mouth.

All around the green lawns and on the forecourt where I was standing, fat pigeons strutted and cooed, and pecked together in peaceful co-existence. I was happy to see them there. I had a fondness for pigeons and their gentle voices. They were welcome to stay so long as they didn't do anything nasty while they were flying over my head or settling on my shoulder. The walls of the whitewashed building were splattered with the nasty things the pigeons had done since the last lot of whitewash was applied. There were extra splatterings beneath the eaves that indicated where the nests were built.

At each of the latticed windows there was a pair of lace curtains drawn closely together as if to discourage Peeping Toms or prying neighbours, and as I looked around I saw one of the curtains twitch, then I caught a glimpse of a head and maybe an inquisitive eye. Soon I was aware that I was being watched by several inquisitive eyes through chinks in the Nottingham lace. Rather reluctantly I turned to go, sad at leaving such a peaceful scene when I had so recently found it.

I had just started to walk away when one of the doors opened and a plump little woman took a short cut across a lawn and hurried over to me. She was wearing a crisply starched wrap-over pinafore that would once have vied with the colourful display on the verandah but was now faded through being put in the wash tub so often. Under the pinny her dress was sprigged with flowers on a more sober background of black. She had a sharp nose and wrinkled cheeks that were faintly flushed with the effort of hurrying. Her snow-white hair was carefully waved and curled with not a strand out of place. She was a very tidy lady.

From behind a pair of National Health spectacles her darting eyes looked me up and down, taking in each detail as they came to it and registering it for future reference. Faced later with a set of Identikit features, she would have unhesitatingly picked out the right ones and put them together to produce a faithful likeness of me.

'Were you looking for somebody, dear?' she asked, still puffing slightly. I suddenly felt conscious of being an intruder.

'No, I was just having a look round, I hope you didn't mind.'

'Of course not, dear,' she said, smiling broadly. 'You wouldn't by any chance be the new matron we're supposed to be getting next month, would you dear?'

Since there seemed no point in making a mystery of it I admitted I was. She threw a swift glance over her shoulder at the latticed windows. There was a hint of triumph in the glance that suggested she was chalking up a victory against those who were frantically twitching their curtains, by being the first to greet the new matron even if I hadn't yet taken up residence.

'Well now, isn't that nice,' she said. 'I just happen to have put the kettle on. Perhaps you'd care for a cup of tea if you're in no particular hurry?'

Since I was in no particular hurry, and because I suspected that she had put the kettle on with me in mind, I said I would like that very much. We walked at a leisurely pace across the grass and alongside the verandah. I noticed several curtains on the lower floor falling into place as we passed them.

The room I was taken to was small and very hot. A fire in the old-fashioned grate burned as fiercely as if there had been a foot of snow outside instead of the bright warmth of a summer's day. The old lady bustled across and poked it afresh, sending sparks flying up the chimney.

'I should undo your cardigan if I were you,' she said, drawing up a chair and inviting me to sit down. 'You won't feel the benefit when you get out if you sit with it buttoned up.' She went off to make the tea and I unbuttoned my cardigan.

It had been something of a disappointment when I was told at one of the interviews that I wouldn't need to wear uniform in my role as matron. I had rather fancied myself in a frilly bonnet with lacy bows, a matronly dress with a touch of lace at neck and cuffs, and maybe even a bunch of keys dangling at my waist. Except for the bunch of keys, all the matrons I had known had worn splendidly regal outfits; not to do so seemed a denial of the title. But now I was glad of it. Long sleeves and a high collar would have sent me reeling out in search of a cooling breeze. I had enough hot flushes already without inviting others by being over-dressed.

I looked round the room. It was bright with flowers. There were flowers on the chenille-covered dining table, flowers on the whatnot, and flowers on the bamboo table beside the single bed that was half concealed by a pair of dividing curtains. There were flowers on every shelf of the built-in dresser, which was the only piece of furniture in the flatlets that didn't belong to the residents. Everything else was theirs, carefully unloaded off the removal van the day they were admitted. This, with the collection of keepsakes, the family portraits and the variety of treasured ornaments, gave to each of the tiny flats its own identity. I was often to be amazed how a fresh set of knick-knacks and a few different pictures on the walls and mantelpiece could transform a room that was basically identical to all the others.

Stretched between two walls of the room where I

was sitting was a length of string on which was pegged another profusion of flowers. It was only when I noticed this that I realized that every bloom in the room was plastic. Plastic nasturtiums trailed from plastic plaited pots, plastic roses climbed out of plastic silver rose bowls and plastic chrysanthemums stood sturdily in plastic Grecian urns. If they hadn't been so dead some of them might have looked quite lifelike.

The old lady came in with the tea and looked apologetically at the wall-to-wall floral display.

'You'll have to excuse the line,' she said, pouring milk into cups. 'I'd have taken them down if I'd known you'd be dropping in, but it's Monday, you see, and they're drying off. I always give them a rinse on Mondays when I've finished me washing. They tend to gather dust if they don't get rinsed regular, and if there's anything I hate to see it's a dusty flower.'

I smiled and nodded to let her know that I was in complete agreement with her sentiments. Then I gently touched a realistic-looking spray of lily-of-the-valley that dangled from the line. It fell at my feet. While I was pegging it back into place between a bunch of variegated polyanthus and some violet-coloured violets, I carelessly dislodged several more bunches and sprays of fragrant blooms, all of which owed whatever fragrance they had to the particular brand of washing powder that had been used to give them their regular Monday rinse. I noticed while I was doing the necessary adjustments that there wasn't a speck of dust on leaf or petal. Each flower was as fresh as a daisy drenched by an April shower.

'There now, that's that then, dear,' said my hostess when we were at last settled at the table with a cup of tea in front of us. There was also a very large vase of plastic gladioli in front of us which rather obstructed our view. The old lady pushed it slightly to one side. One of the gladdies fell out of the vase, obstinately refusing to cooperate when I tried to push it back. 'So you're to be our new matron, are you?' She rose from her chair and stood almost to attention in front of me.

'Pleased to meet you I'm sure, dear,' she said holding out her hand in a very formal way. 'I'm Mrs Turgoose, Polly to me friends.'

I stood up and shook the offered hand. 'I'm very pleased to meet you,' I said and gave her my name in exchange for hers. A single orchid fell off the line.

Looking back later on the introduction ceremony it occurred to me that Mrs Turgoose – Polly to her friends – hadn't shown much interest in the name I gave her. This didn't surprise me as much as it would have done had I not been a nurse. I was used to being nameless on a professional level. Until the day that hospital personnel took to wearing labels telling all and sundry who they were, the patients hadn't thought of them as people with names like anybody else. A nurse was a nurse, a sister a sister, and a matron unmistakably a matron. Occasionally a little confusion arose when a doctor was mistaken for a porter or a senior for a junior, but an icy stare from the doctor or the senior was usually enough to clarify the situation. If it was the porter or the junior who had been elevated to a higher plane, they were content to let the error stay uncorrected. There had been no labels when I was doing my training. Name-dropping then was more selective. I have known malingerers and hypochondriacs be in the same ward for years without ever knowing the sister's surname. Her first name was even more of a dark secret. It would never have done to let the juniors know her name was Dierdre; such a disclosure would have robbed her of the respect she had worked so hard to win, or so it was thought in those days.

Over the tea I learned a great deal about Mrs Turgoose. She had lived in her flat for a long time and was one of the oldest residents. She was very proud of this. From the way she spoke of others who were younger I got the impression that she regarded anybody under seventy as immature. She was also scornful about those who had departed this life prematurely. By prematurely I gathered she meant a decade or two after they had reached the three score years and ten to which they were officially entitled.

'It's stamina you need to keep you going,' she told me after she had run through a list of old friends who had popped off prematurely. 'Without stamina you might just as well be dead. Take my old dad for instance. He'd got stamina. He'd have been a hundred and twenty if he'd lived till Sunday. And what's more, he had all his facilities right to the end.' I was rather glad that he hadn't lived till Sunday, even with all his facilities intact. It turned out that he had died at the respectable age of ninety-nine, sadly just missing getting a telegram from the Queen.

'How old are you?' I asked Mrs Turgoose. I knew I was on safe ground asking the question. The older the elderly are the more they like being asked their age and the more prone they are to adding a year or two. The middle-aged take a year or two off, foolishly expecting to be believed. I did it myself, so I know.

'I'm nearing eighty and good for a bit longer yet I hope,' she said. I looked at her trim little figure, her neatly waved hair and the bright eyes behind the National Health spectacles and said that she looked in good enough shape to beat her father's record. She simpered prettily.

'How old do you have to be before you can come and live here?' I asked, thinking that if all the rooms were occupied by ladies who were nearing their eighties the family doctor must be in great demand, unless they were as healthy as Mrs Turgoose. I waited a little anxiously for her reply. She kept me waiting while she went and got another cup of tea, and put a few more lumps of coal on the fire.

'You had to be at least seventy at one time,' she said, 'but things are different now. There's some in here as isn't a day over sixty-five, still wet behind the ears as you might say. I know for a fact that one of them that's just come in isn't even sixty-five until next week.' She paused for a moment to let the enormity of the crime sink in. 'And what's more, when I first came you had to have belonged to the town all your life before they'd let you in. Nowadays there's Cockneys and all sorts round here.' She sounded as disapproving of Cockneys and all sorts as she was about youngsters of sixty-five, still wet behind the ears.

'But you like living here, don't you?' I said. She looked pensive for a moment and smoothed down her pinny.

'Yes, I like it here all right,' she said at last. 'But it's not the same as it used to be.'

'Why not?' I asked.

'It's never been the same since they started white-washing it and calling it a fancy name. It never used to be whitewashed. It was always a brick colour. And they call it the Lodge now which makes me laugh. They'll never get me to call it that, nor anybody else unless they never knew it by its old name.' She looked very put out.

'What was it called before they started calling it the Lodge?' I asked, thinking of the two men on the road who hadn't known what I was talking about when I mentioned the name.

'As I recall it wasn't called anything,' she said, giving one of the gladdies a push. 'We just used to call it the charities, after them as runs it. You used to have to be poor to get in here you see. Not like some as shall be nameless who came in not short of a bob or two.' From the baleful look she threw at the nameless pluto-crats on the other side of her lace curtains I guessed that she was chronically short of a bob or two which gave us something in common. 'And not only did you have to be poor, you were supposed to be respectable as well. Not all of us were, mind you, but so long as you didn't let the charities know too much when you applied to come in, and could get a parson or some-body to help you fill in the forms and give you a bit of a reference, it was usually only a matter of going on the waiting list and keeping your fingers crossed that somebody would pop off soon and leave a room empty. Mind you, you could wait a long time if them that was in here had as much stamina as my old dad.' She sighed and looked glum. 'But it's not the same as it was. I remember the days when we could have a drop of gin and a knees-up when it was anybody's birthday, or at Christmas and times like that. There's none of that these days. It's all sitting round the fire keeping yourself to yourself and waiting for the parson to call, if you know what I mean. There's even some that goes to church every Sunday.' She sighed deeply, saddened at the thought of such blatant back-sliding in a place once noted for its spirited knees-ups.

'Why can't you have a drop of gin and all the rest of it now when it's anybody's birthday?' I asked, anxious to know where the good times went. Mrs Turgoose bridled angrily.

'It was the matron that was here before the one that's just retired that put the damper on things. She was one of them that can't stand the sight of anybody enjoying themselves. There's some as can't, you know, especially if they've not had too much enjoyment themselves or if they've got themselves too tied up in religion. It's a funny thing about religion. You'd think it would make people happy, but they go round with such long faces that it puts you off. That's why I don't get mixed up in it. That old matron I was telling you about was religious. It was her that got poor old Sal chucked out.'

'Who was she and why did she get chucked out?' I asked, too interested in the things I was hearing to worry about sounding nosy.

'Sal came here the same time as I did. We'd lived next door to each other for years. She got chucked out because she was fond of a drop of gin. She'd been fond of a drop for as long as I'd known her. She never got helpless or anything like that, she just used to sing when she'd had a few. Nothing nasty. "Down by the Old Bull and Bush" and "Nelly Dean" and things like that. But the matron didn't like it. She told Sal that if she didn't mend her ways she'd report her to the charities. Sal was too old to mend her ways so she got reported and they chucked her out. We put in a petition about it, but she had to go. Everybody was up in arms about it, I don't mind telling you.'

'What happened to her after she went?' I asked, trying to shake off the sadness of it all.

'She went to live with one of her sons but he had a la-di-da wife who didn't like Sal singing any more than the matron had, so she didn't reign there long. In the end they put her in one of them places where you sit looking at each other all the time. I went to see her once but she didn't know me so I never went again. The next thing we heard she was dead. I blame that old cow of a matron. Sal might have been here today if she hadn't got chucked out.'

We sat in respectful silence for a moment thinking of poor dead Sal. Then I started to look on the brighter side of things. However sorry I might have felt for Sal and however much I regretted her passing, I felt rather relieved that I wouldn't have to be responsible for someone as fond of a drop as she was. I knew I would be better able to cope with those who kept themselves to themselves and sat waiting for the vicar to call.

After Mrs Turgoose had told me enough about her neighbours past and present to make them turn in their graves or have her sued for slander, I thanked her for the tea and said how nice it had been to make her acquaintance. She stood waving to me from the cardinal red step of her front door and I gave a friendly little wave in the direction of the closely curtained windows but nobody waved back from there.

I had a quick look at the house that was soon to be mine and saw workmen with pots of paint, planks of old wood, planks of new wood, and other things that would make it if not a mansion at least a home. Then I went on my way.

Looking back on the morning it seemed that I would have to be more than just a nurse in my new job. I would need a good pair of ears, the patience to listen and enough wit to appreciate the things I heard. I hoped I would fall short of none of these requirements.

Chapter Three

THE HOUSE THAT I moved into when the workmen moved out wasn't very big. None of its five rooms, three up, two down not counting the kitchen, could have been described as spacious. Neither was it modern. The newest things about it were the floorboards which had been laid in a hurry before I moved in, to get rid of the old ones that had been attacked by rising damp or dry rot. The smell of mildew was everywhere. It seeped into clothing, permeated books and clung to curtains. It embarrassed me by rising from the gloves I wore when I went to church and the handkerchief I took out when I wept at weddings. 'Ah, the Lodge,' breathed family and friends when all they remembered of it was the smell that haunted my belongings.

The bathroom and its accompaniments had been added long after the house was built. It was on the ground floor, jutting out in conspicuous newness from the end wall of the tiny kitchen. Having it there was a mixed blessing. Though it ensured that I didn't have to run upstairs every time I needed to wash my hands in the daytime, it also meant that I had to run downstairs if I needed to wash my hands during the night. This could be a distinct disadvantage in times of stress.

The main feature of the rather dark little house was the number of cupboards and recesses there were in the downstairs rooms. Ants, spiders and silverfish lived in the cupboards and mice chased each other across the recesses. I was never without some sort of wildlife to wage war against. I spent money I could ill afford on insect sprays, and my cheese bills were always heavy.

The three rooms upstairs were reached by a steep and narrow staircase. Each of the rooms was big enough for visiting grandchildren, and their parents as well, to sleep in, and for this alone I was happy to stalk the insects and feed the mice. The joy of having three bedrooms all of my very own offset the cost of the sprays and cheese, especially after I had come so close to having to live in a nurses' home.

There was a very small garden outside the kitchen door. I was glad it wasn't any bigger. If I had never claimed to be a born nurse then neither was I able to boast that I'd got green fingers. Bulbs that I planted deep in the warm brown earth had a tendency to stay there for ever and plants that were dibbled in at the correct depth according to the textbooks shrivelled and died through lack of nourishment or over-feeding. I tried not to look at the garden next door which was lovingly tended by a lady whose every finger was as green as her grass.

On the day that I moved into my new home the little plot was ablaze with summer flowers, a legacy from the previous tenant who also had a full set of green fingers. It looked almost as colourful as Mrs Turgoose's flat. Non-plastic pansies raised their eyebrows to the sun and real live nasturtiums fell from walls and fences in a red and orange glow. The ginger cat that I had first seen sprawled beneath two trees outside my garden was now peacefully sleeping under an apple tree which I could call my own. The apple tree showed signs of a plentiful crop and in its boughs two pigeons and a thrush were preening themselves. I was well content with all I saw.

Between two rows of pretty-faced pansies a path led to a gate which opened onto the forecourt and from my garden I had an unobstructed view of every latticed window. There had been a great deal of activity at the windows while the removal men were staggering up the path with my household effects. This had made me aware that nothing I did in the garden was likely to escape the notice of at least one pair of eyes. Not once in all the years that I was matron of the Lodge did I take an early morning stroll in my dressing gown; not once did I take advantage of even the most gruelling heat wave and recline under the apple tree with my midriff uncovered. I knew instinctively that those whose eyes were on me wouldn't have approved of the matron baring bits of her body in broad daylight.

When the household effects were more or less where I wanted them and the van-men had gone off to slake their thirst with the tip, I started to put the curtains up. I was living dangerously on a stepladder when I saw the garden gate open and Mrs Turgoose coming up the path. She was carrying a tray.

'It's all right, dear, it's only me,' she called from the kitchen door, which she had managed to open before I got there. 'I've brought you a bit of something to eat. I'm sure you must be starving what with the moving in and all that.' I hadn't realized until she said it that I was. She lifted the cover off a plate and showed me a feast that made my mouth water. I stood aside to let her push her way into the kitchen.

'It's not much, dear,' she said with a great show of false modesty. 'It's only a couple of best loin chops which the butcher charged me the earth for, a few green peas that cost me a fortune and some best Jerseys that nearly broke me back carrying them home.' Her sharp little eyes darted round the kitchen. 'Is the cutlery in here?' she asked, diving into a tea chest that I hadn't unpacked. She emerged with a knife and fork, used the newspaper they were wrapped in for a table cloth, then stood at the table with her arms folded watching me eat.

'That was lovely,' I said, chasing the last costly pea round the plate. 'It was terribly nice of you to think of bringing it.' Mrs Turgoose put the plate and its cover on the tray, screwed the newspaper into a ball and threw it into the fireplace, gave the knife and fork a quick rinse under the cold tap and left them to drain.

'Don't mention it, dear,' she said, a self-righteous smirk spreading across her face. 'It was the least I could do under the circumstances. I'm not one to boast and far be it from me to blow my own trumpet, but I'm a fool to myself when it comes to doing a kindness for others. Not like some across there that's got no thought for anybody but themselves. You mark my words, they'll be glad of a helping hand someday.' I thanked her again, laying great stress on the delicacy of the chops, the tenderness of the peas and the unbeatable flavour of the best Jerseys, then I saw her out and went back to hanging the curtains. The hearty lunch I had eaten plus the fact that one of the curtains had unaccountably shrunk since I first measured it gave me a lot of problems when I got on the stepladder.

I was just considering taking the whole lot down and starting again when the garden gate opened and another lady walked up the path carrying a tray. This time I got to the door before she did.

She was a large lady with a figure which might once have had shape but was now nothing more than several stones of quivering flesh. Her pinafore and the dress that sagged below it were a long way past their best; they were not only frayed at the edges but in the middle and sides as well. She was wearing a pair of canvas shoes which may have been white when she bought them but had become several shades of grey over the years. There were two large slashes in each of them, one for her corns, the other for her bunions. Her stockings hung in folds round her ankles. She was spotlessly clean.

'Wotcher mate,' she said, thrusting a tray under my nose. 'I've brought you a bit of dinner. I thought you'd be feeling peckish seeing as you've been at it all morning.' I relieved her of the tray and thanked her for the generous thought. When I asked her if she would care to step inside she was in like a shot, and looking suspiciously round the kitchen. It was bare except for the tea chests that I hadn't unpacked and one or two that I had.

'That's funny,' she said, opening a cupboard door and disturbing a couple of woodlice. 'I could have sworn I saw Polly Turgoose come over not so long ago carrying a tray or something.' It seemed she had missed Mrs Turgoose's departure with the empties. Hastily I positioned myself between her and the draining board. I didn't want her to be hurt at seeing the knife and fork which would tell her that she was second in what I feared might be a long line of ladies bearing lunches. I detected enough rivalry already between her and Mrs Turgoose without me stirring up more by letting her know that I had eaten well at her enemy's expense.

The liver and onions were lovely. And so were the vegetables. They would no doubt have been even better if I hadn't had my appetite blunted with the substantial first course I'd eaten not half an hour before. I struggled valiantly, closely watched by the cook.

'That was delicious,' I said controlling a burp. 'The liver was quite the best I have ever tasted.'

'It should have been,' she said, 'considering the price

of it.' She put the empty plate and its cover back on the tray but I managed to grab the knife and fork before she walked away with them to the sink.

Just before she went out of the door she said something which made the two meals I had eaten collide inside me with a gentle lurch.

'There was a nice basin of jellied eels in the larder you could have had but I thought you might like the liver best for your dinner. I'll bring the eels across for your tea. See you about five, mate.'

I had never eaten a jellied eel. I wasn't sure that I would be ready for anything so exotic by five o'clock, but before I had time to say so the old lady had shuffled off down the path. Mercifully there were no more lunches that day.

The jellied eels started their journey up the path just as I was thanking Mrs Turgoose for the poached egg on toast and slice of rich fruit cake she kindly brought for my tea. The two ladies met, one leaving, the other arriving. The path was too narrow for them to pass without somebody giving way and in the ensuing encounter the basin of jellied eels landed upside down in a pansy bed. I hurried to the scene hoping to put an end to hostilities before they got out of hand.

By the time I reached them the two ladies were squaring up to each other in a most unladylike way.

Realizing that my aptitude for peacemaking was about to be put to the test, I offered up a quick prayer that the threatened confrontation would confine itself to words and not descend to anything as sordid as blows.

'Oh dear,' I cried looking at the catastrophe in the pansy bed. 'However did they get down there?' Before either of the ladies had time to give me her version of the events that had led to the tragedy, the ginger cat, that had been sleeping under the apple tree, woke, stretched himself, caught a breath of fishy air and swooped. Within seconds there was no trace of jelly or eels.

The three of us had watched their dispatch in silence. We remained silent until the cat had streaked up the apple tree to sit on a branch and wash his whiskers. The lady who had brought the eels was the first to speak.

'Bloody cat,' she said with intense feeling. She picked the basin out of the pansies. 'They should never have let it in the place. It's nothing but a flaming nuisance.'

'That's right,' said Mrs Turgoose, now on the friendliest terms with her enemy. 'There's rules against bringing cats and dogs in here and folks should be made to abide by them. They wouldn't let me bring my dog and he was all I had in the world. He had to go to the vet to be put down and I'd only just had him there to be doctored. It broke my heart, it did.' Tears welled up in her eyes.

The two ladies walked in single file down the path and out of the gate. I let the cat stay in the apple tree. I was grateful to him for making short work of the eels. I should have hated to have to eat them myself. The poached egg on toast and the fruit cake were already warring with the liver and onions and all the other things I had eaten for lunch. An eel going into combat would have upset things beyond the help of Alka-Seltzer.

I also had wondered why the ginger cat had been allowed to take up residence at the Lodge. I knew the rules about keeping pets. They had been explained to me very carefully at one of the interviews. Like most of the other rules that were explained to me, they dated back to the days when the whitewashed building was still brick coloured and hadn't got its fancy name. It had been a philanthropic idea conceived by a man with a great deal of money that he didn't know what to do with. Knowing he couldn't take it with him when he died, he arranged things so that a chosen few of the elderly ladies of reduced circumstances in the town should benefit from it. He also left instructions about rules and regulations. Those who carried out his instructions did so to the letter. They nailed a copy of the rules in every flatlet and warned incoming residents of the penalties of breaking the rules. There was really only one penalty and that was to be chucked out like poor old Sal had been, but as far as I could gather hers was an isolated case. Maybe she wouldn't have been dealt with so harshly if the matron could have brought herself occasionally to join in the chorus of 'Nellie Dean' or 'Down by the Old Bull and Bush'. Even the rowdiest party doesn't sound so bad if you are part of it.

The rule about pets was heavily underscored so that nobody would be left in any doubt of its importance. It clearly stated that no cat, dog, or other animal or any sort of poultry whatsoever should be kept on the premises under any pretence by the occupier. After I had choked back a giggle at the thought of a goat being tethered to a bedpost or a pig tied to a table leg, I asked the man who was interviewing me whether there had ever been such flagrant defiance of the rules.

'It isn't as funny as you seem to think,' he said crossly. 'I could tell you a lot about that place that would surprise you.' He proceeded to tell me something that was just as funny as my vision of the pig and the goat.

According to a story that was buried somewhere in the archives, two of the chosen poor, who were admitted almost as soon as the charitable idea took shape, had been fattening up a goose and a cockerel in the backyards of their old homes, when they heard they were next on the list for a flatlet. Neither of them could bear to think of their Christmas dinner going to waste, so they had smuggled the poultry in, still alive and kicking. Every morning the rooster stretched its neck and announced the dawn, and the goose in the adjoining flat joined in with a raucous screech.

When the rest of the residents grew weary of having their slumbers disturbed at sunrise, they signed a petition with a few names and a lot of crosses, and threatened that unless the nuisance ceased forthwith the petition would go to the committee for them to do their worst. The owner of the cockerel, who wasn't a bad woman at heart, promised to do her best to keep her Christmas dinner quiet. For the next week or two she woke before the cockerel and placed a sack over its head to stop it from having a good crow, which had a soothing effect on the goose as well. But when the sack was left off and the nuisance was committed again the petition was solemnly presented to the committee. They went into conclave and decided that Christmas would have to be a little early that year. They ordered that the goose and the cockerel should be executed at once and a new set of rules was nailed up in every flatlet, with some even heavier underscoring.

'But aren't they allowed to keep a pet at all?' I had asked the man who was interviewing me. I remembered my mother and the dog she had doted on, which in his own special way had made up for some of the emptiness in the house after my father died. I remembered also a cat which a maiden aunt of mine had cherished dearly, though I had never looked on it with any great favour. I was sure that the Lodge would have its share of lonely widows and maiden aunts all desperately needing something to love.

'Well,' he said, clearing his throat as if he was preparing to say something he was slightly ashamed of saying. 'We don't allow cats or dogs to be taken into the Lodge but over the years we have relaxed the rules about budgerigars and other small cage birds. We still exclude parrots, however. One did manage to get in once, but it proved to be just as much of a nuisance as the goose and the cockerel were. Eventually it had to go.'

When the interview was over I had promised faithfully that should my application for the post of matron of the Lodge be successful I would keep a sharp lookout for illegal entries, but turn a blind eye to the smaller feathered friends that arrived in chromium cages. The little birds that I turned a blind eye to were to cause me many a heartache in the coming years. The death of a budgerigar or a singing canary could bring so much desolation to its owner that I was almost as saddened by the bereavement as she was.

Having heard the rules so plainly stated against four-legged friends being allowed in the Lodge, the presence of the ginger cat continued to puzzle me until I heard the story much later of how he had managed to get through the tight security net. It was a story that warmed my heart when I first heard it, but it lost a lot of its pathos after the cat had become a thorn in my flesh.

There were other rules on the list nailed to the kitchen doors that had ceased to have any significance over the years. Insisting that no occupier of any of the flats should take in lodgers may have been a necessary safeguard against overcrowding in the days of Queen Victoria, but with each of the living rooms being only just big enough to accommodate one person in comfort, the danger of any of them becoming a boarding house seemed very remote. Again the man who was interviewing me had wiped the smile off my face. He assured me that it had been known to happen, albeit a long time ago and on a very small scale. He could cite cases he said – in strictest confidence, of course, he being a lawyer – where a brother, a sister who had fallen by the wayside, or a prodigal son who had expected a fatted calf, had been bundled into a flatlet under cover of night and kept hidden like a stowaway until all was discovered. Then somebody from the committee was sent to evict the lodger and warn the erring landlady that the same thing would happen to her if she was ever caught breaking the rules again.

But such things were of the past. Occasionally a visitor, female of course, was allowed to snuggle up in bed beside the regular occupant, but only for a very short visit and after written consent had been obtained from the committee. The charitable body of the day had no more intention of letting the Lodge become a holiday camp than their forefathers had of seeing it degenerate into a doss house for itinerants.

Another of the rules still included in the list, though not as needfully as it might have been in the good old days, was that all applicants for a flatlet should be clean, sober and of good order. Some were more orderly than others but, except for the unfortunate Sally whose insobriety had been her downfall, there was nothing in the records to suggest that any of the residents, either past or present, had reeled up the cul-de-sac in an advanced state of intoxication. Once the drop of gin and the knees-up on festive occasions had been stamped out, respectability reigned and any celebrating was kept strictly within the terms of the rules laid down by the charitable body. Necks got washed regularly and the peace was never breached by high-pitched renderings of 'Nelly Dean' or other songs sacred to soloists who have been on a binge. This was a great relief to those who liked to keep themselves to themselves and had never sung 'Nelly Dean' in their lives, but could be quite inhibiting for others who would have preferred their Christmases and birthdays to be a little less sober, even if they didn't touch a drop at any other time.

One of the first things I had to learn when I became matron of the Lodge was the importance of distinguishing between the two types. It would never have done for me to burst into somebody who had never heard of Becher's Brook with the news that the favourite had fallen at the first fence, neither would it have pleased the frustrated members of the knees-up brigade to be given an account, however brief, of the vicar's sermon that had almost made me nod off in my pew the previous Sunday morning. I learned to gloom a little with those who enjoyed a good gloom, laugh with those to whom laughter came easily, and listen with rapt attention to the story I had heard so often that I could have told it myself without any prompting. I made almost as many mistakes while I was learning as I made when I was learning how to be a nurse.

Chapter Four

THE MATRON WHO had so conveniently reached retiring age just when I was starting to get desperate about my future hadn't lived in the house that went with the job. Being a single lady and having no future grandchildren to plan for, she had chosen to live in one of the flatlets. I had visited her there several times before I officially took her place.

Her name was Miss Bains. She was a gentle lady, tall, slender and with an air of refinement which was sometimes a little awesome. Her flat was a joy to behold. Over the years she had gathered such a collection of small treasures that great care had to be taken not to dislodge any of them. One sweeping gesture in the vicinity of the dresser and a whole set of toby jugs could be put in jeopardy, or a collection of miniature animals become an endangered species. I was very conscious of this when I visited her and kept the gestures to a minimum and never went near the whatnot without exercising the greatest caution. I was given to extravagant gestures when I got carried away.

On the first few occasions that I took tea with her the conversation was kept strictly to business. Miss Bains told me the things she thought I should know about the residents, even including some of their little idiosyncrasies, though not in an unkind way. She mentioned casually that Mrs Turgoose would keep me in touch with the happenings at the Darby and Joan club, and the happenings round the Lodge as well if they were sufficiently startling. She said that little Miss Coombe who lived in the corner was very shy and found it difficult to talk to anybody except her budgerigar. She mentioned Mrs Marsh who I later discovered was the lady who had brought the jellied eels; but it wasn't until a few days before I moved in that she mentioned she was about to get married. This came as much of a shock to me as it had apparently done to the residents. But, being a rather reserved lady, she hadn't gone into any great detail about the forth-coming marriage. It was left to Mrs Turgoose to do that, which she obligingly did on the first Monday morning that I started my duties.

'Fancy her getting tied up at her age,' she said, tossing her head contemptuously and throwing a bunch of Michaelmas daisies into a sink full of suds.

'You'd have thought a woman like her would have had more sense. She kept it under her hat as well. None of us round here knew anything about it until the bans were read out last Sunday. The woman at the end that goes to church came and told us. I don't mind telling you, we were all a bit upset, her not breathing a word to anybody.'

'She's never been married before, has she?' I said, wondering if such a step shouldn't be taken sooner if it was going to be taken at all; though I knew from sad experience that even then there was no guarantee of its being a success.

'No,' replied Mrs Turgoose with a sneer in her voice. 'It's the first time round for her, which in my opinion makes it even dafter.'

'Is it the first time round for him as well?' I asked. Mrs Turgoose rinsed the Michaelmas daisies under the tap and shook them to get the excess water out. I stepped back to avoid being splashed.

'Now that's a different kettle of fish altogether,' she said, taking a peg from a hand-embroidered peg bag. 'She'll be his third or fourth, I'm not sure which. But whichever it is, I've no doubt he'll be able to teach old Bains a thing or two. Him being more experienced so to speak.' She gave me a dig in the ribs that nearly knocked me over.

'Have they known each other long?' I asked, tenderly massaging the place where she'd dug.

'They've known each other since they were at school together, but they've only been what you might call courting since his last wife died a year or two ago. He started bringing her home from chapel on Sunday night and before you could say Jack Robinson she was asking him in for cups of cocoa. It caused a lot of talk round here, as you can imagine.' I could imagine. From the things Mrs Turgoose had told me the first time I met her I already guessed that it would take less than an invitation for cocoa after chapel to cause talk.

I had to wait a little longer before Miss Bains gave me afternoon tea and her version of the romance that hadn't so much burst into her life as seeped into it gradually. She was pink and bubbling. The hand that passed cucumber sandwiches shook slightly; the tea she poured came erratically out of the spout and fell into saucer as well as cup. She was in a highly nervous state.

'Such a dear, kind man,' she murmured of her future intended. 'And such a devoted husband to each of his former wives. I knew them all you see. We were girls together and remained friends even when I left home to do my training. And now he has done me the honour of asking me to be his fourth wife. He has been so lonely since dear Elspeth died.' I took the cup and saucer off her before she dropped them in my lap.

I was delighted to hear that she had been on such good terms with the former wives. I had read letters in the agony columns of women's magazines from ladies who were married to previously married men. Not all the marriages had worked out well. There were sad little stories of comparisons that had been made by husbands whose former wives, according to him, were peerless. If Miss Bains's husband's three former wives had been peerless, she could find herself striving to compete.

But it sounded as if she had already faced up to this and was more than willing to live with the ghosts of the past. None the less, I felt it my duty to warn her of one or two pitfalls.

'You'll lose your independence,' I said, thinking of the years she had been single, and free to read in bed for as long as she liked without somebody wanting the light turned off; and the dainty little meals she ate at times to suit herself; the meals would have to be bigger and the times mightn't suit a man. She laughed and shook her head.

'I've had my independence for more than sixty years, I shall be quite happy to lose at least some of it – if indeed I have to.'

'But what if he gets ill?' I persisted, remembering that the man we were talking about was several years her senior. She laughed again.

'If he gets ill I shall nurse him,' she replied, with such assurance that I gave up trying to spoil the best thing that had ever happened to her, and began instead to decide whether she should wear a dove-grey suit or a rose-pink dress and jacket on her wedding day. We finally settled for the dove-grey suit; it would be more practical for wearing on occasions after the main event.

I took an afternoon off later in the week and went with her to buy the last-minute things for her trousseau. She went quite pink when she told me she still hadn't bought any nightwear.

'I've always worn pyjamas,' she said in a low voice so that the girl who was waiting to serve us wouldn't hear. 'I found them so much more convenient when one of the residents rang her emergency bell in the night. And warmer too. But possibly a nightdress might be more appropriate under the circumstances.' She blushed again.

I said that since she wouldn't be getting up in the night to answer emergency bells I thought she could safely discard the pyjamas in favour of something more feminine. We chose one nightdress in blue with ecru lace at neck and wrist, another in peach and another in a very pale mauve.

The wedding was attended by the groom's many sons and daughters, their children, and their children's children. I sat at the back of the chapel with several of the ladies from the Lodge and we whispered together about the bride's dove-grey outfit, the groom's old-fashioned morning suit and the look of frailty he wore while he was getting married.

When the service was over and the children's children had presented them with things to bring them luck, we threw a little confetti; then we all went to a select place in the town for champagne and a buffet lunch, after which the bride and groom were driven off in a car bedecked with ribbons. It was all done with great ceremony and Miss Bains's new husband hadn't looked blasé about any of it. In fact, he became so flushed with happiness after his second glass of champagne that some of us wondered whether it had been too much for him, and even expressed doubts that he would get as far as Brighton where it was rumoured they were honeymooning. I was standing next to Mrs Turgoose when their car turned the corner.

'Ah well, that's that then, dear,' she said, brushing confetti off the front of her coat. 'I must say he looked quite chirpy once they got him in the car. Let's hope he can keep it up, at least until the honeymoon's over. It'd be a shame if old Bains came home not much wiser than she was when she went, if you get my meaning like.' She dug an elbow into my ribs.

I wasn't sure if I wanted to get her meaning. I had always thought of marriage between two people of a more mature age to be the union of minds rather than having any physical significance. But when I hinted at this to Mrs Turgoose she gave me a withering look.

'Don't you believe it, dear,' she said. 'The only difference when you're getting on a bit, if you're still interested, is that you get a longer ride for your money, neither of you being in the first flush so to speak.' I moved away quickly.

Marriage seemed to suit Miss Bains. Whenever I met her in the town, and on the occasions that she invited me to her rather grand house for tea, she was blooming. Being her husband's fourth time round didn't appear to have blunted his capacity for making her happy. Anything else it may have blunted was a matter of concern for them alone but Mrs Turgoose made it hers too. I was black and blue round the ribs before Miss Macintosh, who lived in an upstairs flat, gave her and everybody else something else to think about.

The news of Miss Macintosh's sudden change of fortune was brought to me by Mrs Marsh who lived immediately below her. As well as being the lady whose jellied eels had come to such a sad end, Mrs Marsh was one of the Cockneys Mrs Turgoose had mentioned when she was telling me about the foreigners who had started to invade the Lodge. Anybody not born within the sound of the parish church bells was a foreigner to Mrs Turgoose. Mrs Marsh had been born within the sound of Bow bells, which not only made her a foreigner but put her in a very poor light with those, like Mrs Turgoose, who didn't understand the language.

After the Blitz had robbed Mrs Marsh of nearly everything she possessed in the world, which wasn't much, she came to live with one of her sons in the comparative safety of our town. She hadn't liked it at all. Nothing her son did for her ever made up for her old way of life in the street that was bombed. She was a stranger in a strange land; an exile, fifteen miles from home, surrounded by people who, however much pity they felt for the blitzed, found it hard to integrate. They also found it hard to accept the tattered dress and pinny, and the slashed-up shoes which Mrs Marsh didn't bother to change when she popped up the street for a bottle of Guinness.

'Bloody snobs,' she said to her son when the neighbours tried not to look down at the shabby shoes, and hurried by when Mrs Marsh would have liked to stop for a chat.

None of Mrs Marsh's old neighbours would have hurried by. They had stood in little groups outside shop doors or outside their front doors often for the best part of a morning or afternoon having lovely chats. And they had all worn shabby shoes, except for the time when the shoe shop in the next street was bombed; then everybody had rushed round after the dust had settled and helped themselves. The copper who came and caught them let them off with a caution, and pretended not to see the bulges under their coat or in the pockets where the shoes were stuffed. Only if there were too many bulges did he take action.

Mrs Marsh and her neighbours had always been poor. But before the war came to spoil things they had been able to forget their poverty on Saturday nights. For the price of a drop of gin or a jug or two of ale there was dancing and singing, and friendship unlimited in the pub on the corner. Even the policeman who had steered Mrs Marsh home at closing time was as good as a son to her. 'Goodnight, Ma, sleep tight,' he'd say as he pushed her into her front door. And sleep tight she did, tighter than she slept while the war was on and for a long time after it ended.

All this she told me and a lot more besides while I was sitting holding her hand after she'd rung for me in the night when she had had one of her bad dreams.

'Listen,' she would say, clutching my hand in terror, 'there's another of them going over. We'd better get down to the shelter quick before they blow our bloody heads off.' She had seen a woman get her head blown off when a bomb fell at her feet and the horror was to stay with her for the rest of her life. It took time for me to convince her that the war was over and that bombs and air-raid shelters were things of the past, and when I had she would doze again, only to wake with a start when another Messerschmitt droned through her dreams. I spent a lot of time holding Mrs Marsh's hand when I should have been enjoying a good night's rest.

It was easy to see that Mrs Marsh wasn't the house-proud woman that Mrs Turgoose was. No well-rinsed plastic flowers were pegged out on wash days and there were no neat covers spread over the loose covers that kept the original upholstery clean. Mrs Turgoose's uncut moquette hadn't seen the light of day since it was delivered many years ago from the spot-cash furniture shop. It was protected from the laying on of unclean hands or any other part of the anatomy, and also from fading, by layer after layer of easily removable slipovers which were washed as regularly as the plastic flowers.

Mrs Marsh's settee and two armchairs didn't have any covers at all. The Rexine three-piece suite was already on its last legs when it was haggled for on the pavement outside a junk shop near enough to a bus stop for the waiting queue to relax for a moment on the thoughtfully provided seats. A badly sprung bed, a table and a mat or two had also been haggled for, and these, with an odd assortment of jumble-sale bargains, were all she had. She wouldn't have had those if her son and the rest of her family hadn't had a whip-round to buy them. They had previously had a bonfire with the worm-eaten bits and pieces she had brought with her from London which were salvaged from the wreckage. She told me that it had brought tears to her eyes to see the last links with her past being reduced to ashes in her son's back garden. It brought tears to my eyes as well, but I wasn't sure if I was laughing or crying. I never did when Mrs Marsh was telling me her little stories. She had a way of putting things which made me either fall about in mild hysteria or weep in sympathy with her tears. Occasionally I got the two mixed up.

Her husband had been a humper in Smithfield market. He died young. According to Mrs Marsh, he had a heart of gold when he was sober though a bit free with his fists after he'd had a few, which was every Saturday night. But he had been a good father, she said, and that, coupled with the fuss he made of her after he had finished thumping her, more than compensated for the bruises. Time had dimmed the memory of the poverty-stricken miseries she had endured in those early days and she had a soft light in her eyes even when she was telling me about the thumpings. One of the most spectacular of these had been her reward for pawning her husband's best trousers on the very day that he wanted to wear them.

'He only used to wear them at weekends,' she told me one night when she was too frightened to go to sleep. 'Every Monday morning I would nip them round to the pop shop and fetch them out again on Friday after he'd given me the housekeeping money. I'd been doing it ever since we were married and he'd never twigged. Then one Monday night there was this humpers' meeting or something and he turned the house upside down looking for his best trousers. I had to sneak out the back door and run up the street to ask a mate of mine to lend me a tanner to get them out. But when I got home he'd rumbled me. He stuck his hand in one of the pockets and brought out half-a-crown. He'd been meaning to give it me on me birthday he said, but he gave me a bloody good hiding instead, then went off to the meeting and came home helpless. He'd spent my birthday money and nearly ruined his best trousers. He was a fine man, was my Harry.'

Mrs Marsh had never paid spot cash for anything that she could get with a small down payment and some very irregular weekly instalments. Almost from the day she got married hordes of worried tally men had rushed to be the first at her door on Monday mornings before the housekeeping money ran out. They often had to wait on the step while she went to borrow the money she owed them from somebody she had lent it to the week before. This was such a regular performance that there was always some confusion in the street about which money belonged to which neighbour. The confusion sometimes led to high words or even a black eye.

'Folks aren't like that these days,' she said sadly when she was reminiscing over the monetary system which had kept her and her neighbours out of the debtors' prison. 'Trying to borrow a bob is like getting blood from a stone, especially round here. It's not like it used to be in London, where nobody had much but they was always willing to share it with those who had less.'

There were other things which Mrs Marsh missed after she left London, and continued to miss after she came to live at the Lodge. She would shuffle along the verandah in her frayed pinafore and canvas shoes, looking wistfully at the windows hoping that somebody would see her through the curtains and invite her in for a chat. But few ever did. Those who kept themselves to themselves were kind but distant when they saw her, and even those who at first showed a willingness to be friendly soon grew tired of seeing her standing on their step with an empty cup in her hand asking for the loan of a bit of sugar until she could get to the shops to buy some. She had long since stopped asking for the loan of a bob or two. Being short of a shilling got her no more invitations to go in for a chat than running out of sugar.

When she realized that none of the ploys she used to gain entrance was working, she put on an old tweed coat over the pinafore and went off to the town, hoping to meet somebody who wasn't too stuck up to talk to her; or she dropped in at one of the old folk's clubs and upset the regular members by arguing with them. The reason she argued with them was because she didn't much care for the elderly who frequented clubs for the elderly. She thought they were snobs and made it her business to tell them so, which didn't improve her chances of being made welcome. She stopped darkening the doors of the old folk's clubs after she wasn't chosen to be Dowager Queen of the Borough in the first year that the Borough had a Dowager Queen. The little woman who was given the honour had not only lived in the town all her life but had never been known to go to the club wearing a pinafore. She would be every inch a Dowager Queen.

'Bloody favouritism,' stormed Mrs Marsh when she was telling me how the voting went. 'They only picked her out because she's well in with the warden. I shouldn't be a bit surprised if the ballot was rigged.' I felt sorry for her, knowing how she had set her heart on being Dowager Queen, but I couldn't quite see her in a sequined gown and gilt-encrusted crown opening a supermarket.

The day she brought me news of Miss Macintosh's brief rise to fame if not to fortune, she steamed up the garden path and burst through my back door, not waiting for me to open it for her.

'That Miss Macintosh in the flat above me has had a man in her room,' she gasped after I had sat her in a chair before she collapsed at my feet. She wasn't built for hurrying and she must have hurried quite fast up the path.

'Well, and what if she has?' I asked coldly. 'There's nothing in the rules that says you can't have a man in your room, is there?'

'Maybe there isn't,' said Mrs Marsh. 'But there's men and men, and the one that went up to Miss Macintosh wasn't your ordinary sort of man.'

'What sort was he?' I asked. I knew I shouldn't have asked but I told myself that if there was a special sort of man hanging about and visiting the residents it was my duty as matron to find out more about him. He could have been a burglar – or even a murderer. I refused to admit that it was sheer curiosity that made me ask.

'Well he had a bowler hat on for a start, which not many men wear these days. And he'd got one of them satchels that office chaps use to carry their sandwiches in. He wasn't a tally man or anything like that, I know them all as comes round here. And it wasn't an insurance man either. They come on bikes and never look very well off. This bloke was in a car and he looked a lot better off than you or me. She's a dark horse is that Macintosh woman. It wouldn't surprise me if she's up to something. Still waters run deep as they say.'

It would have surprised me very much if Miss Macintosh had been up to something in the way that Mrs Marsh seemed to be implying. She was Scottish and had such a delightful accent that when she told me she came from the Bridge of Earn I begged her to say it again. She made it sound like music. Still waters and a dark horse she may have been, but nothing she did or had ever done could have been less than rigidly honest.

I let Mrs Marsh tell me all she could about the man with the satchel and bowler hat, then I sternly reminded her that since it was none of her business or mine either it would be better if she went home and stopped tittle-tattling. After she had gone I sat and racked my brains to think who Miss Macintosh's visitor might have been. I knew that she had no family except a distant cousin who lived abroad and whom she hadn't seen for years. Her friends could be counted on one hand and didn't include the sort of man that Mrs Marsh had described. Whoever it was must have had some very good reason for coming. I hoped that Mrs Marsh wouldn't be too long finding out more. She was back within the hour.

'It was the law,' she said, falling into a chair that had once been my mother's and which was just the right height for breathless old ladies to fall into. 'Not one of them from the cop shop, more of a lawyer like them on the charities committee.'

'How on earth did you find out?' I asked. I knew

that Miss Macintosh wasn't the sort to pour out her life story to Mrs Marsh, though she would occasionally fill the empty cup with sugar. She had a kind heart as well as a lovely Scottish accent.

'To tell you the truth I played a bit of a trick on her,' said Mrs Marsh giving me a sly look. 'His car was still there after I left you, so I hung about until he came down, then I went up as fast as I could and knocked at her door. She thought it was him as had forgotten something and I was in before she had time to shut it again.'

'Well, I think that was a disgusting thing to do,' I said, shocked to the core. 'And what happened then?'

'I said I'd seen a strange man going up the stairs and was worried in case she'd come to any harm, or if he'd come to bring her bad news.'

'And what did she say?'

'She didn't say much, her being a dark horse, but as far as I could make out the bloke had come to tell her that somebody who lives in foreign parts has died and left her a fortune. It's a funny thing that nobody ever dies and leaves me a fortune. It's them what 'as gets, as they say.' Nobody had ever died and left me a fortune nor was ever likely to.

'Did she tell you how much she'd been left?' I asked, allowing curiosity to triumph over discretion.

'No, but it must have been a tidy sum for her to have mentioned it at all. You know how tight lipped she can be, and tight fisted as well sometimes, though she will set me at liberty with a bit of sugar when I'm down to my last grain, which is more than some of them will round here.'

My visitor looked as if she was prepared to sit all day speculating on the size of Miss Macintosh's fortune but I had heard enough. I again reminded her that it was none of our business and the less she said about it the better. By the look on her face when she went out of the door I knew she could hardly wait to spread the news to the largest number of people in the shortest possible time. Long before nightfall the Lodge was buzzing with speculation about the heiress.

It wasn't until I did the first round the following morning that I saw Miss Macintosh. She looked no different than she always did. She had obviously recovered from the shock of becoming suddenly so rich. We went through the usual pattern of my routine visits, inquiring politely after each other's health, mentioning what terrible weather it had been lately and touching briefly on the television programme we had watched the previous evening. Then just as I was edging towards the door knowing no more than I already knew, she relented.

'If you've a minute to spare there's something I'd like to tell you,' she said. I sat down, tingling with anticipation.

'I had a caller yesterday who brought me some news.' I tried to look as if it was the first I'd heard about the caller.

'I hope it was good news,' I said. She looked surprised.

'But surely Mrs Marsh came over and told you,' she said innocently. I blushed. She had obviously watched Mrs Marsh's second journey up the path.

'Actually, she did come and tell me she'd dropped in to see you.' The blush spread as Miss Macintosh gazed at me. There was a twinkle in her eyes.

'She dropped in to find out all she could about the man who visited me,' she said. 'I'm afraid I rather misled her. She went away believing that I had come into a great deal of money.' The blush turned into a hot flush that spread a long way down my neck. I took out a handkerchief and patted my burning face. I remembered with shame how easily I had been led to believe what Mrs Marsh had told me.

'What news did your caller bring?' I asked, realizing that Miss Macintosh was waiting for the question. She looked sad for a moment.

'It concerned the cousin I told you about who lived

abroad and whom I haven't seen for years. She died recently and left a great deal of money. Since I hadn't seen her for such a long time the news of her death wasn't too distressing.' She paused and waited for me to put the next question to her. I wasn't quite sure how to do it.

'Then – er.' I stopped. 'That means then that you are – er.' I stopped again.

'If you are trying to ask me whether I've become rich overnight the answer is no. I'm not a penny better off than I was before.' The mischievous look came back. 'The only thing my cousin left me was a very old family Bible, though I'm afraid I didn't make that clear to Mrs Marsh. I'm dreadfully afraid that she jumped to quite the wrong conclusion.' I dabbed at my face again with the handkerchief.

'But if she didn't leave her fortune to you, then who did she leave it to?' I asked, made bold by her mischievous look. She burst out laughing.

'She left the lot to a donkey sanctuary,' she spluttered. 'Every penny of it. She had always had a great fondness for donkeys and she knew I wouldn't want it, I have enough for my needs. Now you see why I couldn't possibly have told Mrs Marsh the whole story. She would never have believed it.' I hardly believed it myself. I sat for a moment thinking of all that money being used to make donkeys happy, then I burst out laughing myself.

It was a while before rumours about the heiress died down. Some of the residents stood at their windows watching for trappings of wealth to be delivered to Miss Macintosh's flat, but when nothing happened they lost interest. Soon it was only Mrs Marsh who mentioned it. She found it hard to forgive Miss Macintosh for being rich. She was particularly bitter after she had climbed the stairs with an empty cup and climbed down again with the cup still empty.

'How anybody can be so mean I'll never know,' she said after one of these fruitless journeys. 'If it was me that had come into all that money I'd be only too glad to set somebody at liberty with a bit of sugar, or even a bob or two now and again. She didn't even open the door when I knocked.'

'Perhaps she's out,' I said. Mrs Marsh shook her head.

'No, it's like all them millionaires, they don't like to part with it. And what I'd like to know is what she thinks will happen to it when she goes. She can't take it with her and she's got nobody belonging to her so what's she hoarding it for?'

'She'll probably leave it to a home for cats or a

donkey sanctuary,' I said. Mrs Marsh gave me a dirty look and then she laughed.

'Nobody would be daft enough to do a thing like that,' she cackled.

Part Two

Chapter Five

BECAUSE OF THE ruling that those on the waiting list for one of the flatlets should have lived in the town for at least two years, most of the applicants were known by those already in residence. A great deal of speculation went on about who would move in when there was a vacancy. Rumours were rife. There were whisperings in the church, in chapel, at the old people's clubs and at whist drives. Names were mentioned and hopes raised. Though no money changed hands there were hot tips passed round by those who declared they had got their information from the highest source. They never disclosed the source.

Sometimes the forecasting on who was next in line for admission turned out to be accurate, but more often than not it was wide of the mark. The charitable body allowed no leaks to spoil the surprise.

When Miss Bains got married and moved out of her grace-and-favour flatlet there was the usual excitement. The ones who got their information from the highest source said that without doubt the next tenant would be Mrs Clarke who had fallen on hard times when her husband, who everybody thought was rich, had died and left her penniless. Those who were only guessing said that in their opinion it had to be old Mrs Topliss who had scrubbed the church for forty-five years and would still have been scrubbing it but for the fact that she had started leaving her bucket and mop in the aisle for the unwary to trip over when they went in for a quick prayer before the lights were turned on.

The reason that nobody had mentioned Mrs Beauchamp was because nobody knew her. She had lived in the town much longer than the statutory two years but on the south side and out of reach of the forecasters.

On the day she arrived heads popped out of doors and eyes peeped out of windows. Mrs Marsh found to her amazement that she had run out of sugar and wandered along the verandah with a cup in her hand; Mrs Turgoose puffed up the stairs to visit her friend Mrs Smythe, who had a commanding view of the forecourt from her window; and Miss Coombe, who had a reputation for keeping herself to herself, actually came out and had a word with Mrs Marsh.

The new arrival made a splendid entry. There was a

style about it which made me almost wish that I was wearing the full regalia of a matron instead of a skirt and a hand-knitted twin-set. Since I had knitted them both, neither the jumper nor the cardigan was flawless.

I was often afflicted by the same lack of confidence when visitors who hadn't been to the Lodge before stopped and asked me where they could find the matron. They always seemed surprised when I told them they already had. No matter how much I tried to boost my own morale by reminding myself that in spite of appearances I was a State Registered Nurse and a matron to boot, there were times when I would have benefited greatly from some outward and visible proof. One of these times was when Mrs Beauchamp came to live amongst us.

I waited until the portly middle-aged man had heaved himself out of his car and had helped his mother to disentangle herself from the rugs, then I straightened my skirt, pulled in my tummy muscles and stepped nervously forward to greet them. They stood side by side in a way that suggested they expected a red carpet to be unrolled at their feet. I forestalled the question that I saw trembling on the portly gentleman's lips by telling him that I was the matron. He seemed taken aback; not so his mother. She said how delighted she was to meet me, then threw her arms round me and embraced me warmly. Remembering my own mother who, when she was roughly the same age as Mrs Beauchamp, had greeted strangers with the enthusiasm usually reserved for closer acquaintances, I knew at once that the newcomer was very much to my liking.

Mrs Beauchamp was small and slim, and pretty in a soft and kittenish way. She wore her clothes with an air that disguised the fact that they had seen better days. It was only when I knew her better that I discovered she had a knack of throwing on any old rag and making it look more elegant than another woman's newly bought creation. The woolly caps she invariably wore sat beautifully on her head and she could do things with a scarf that transformed the oldest and simplest dress into high fashion. I envied her the knack. A woolly cap looked like a tea cosy whichever way I wore it and I only had to tie a scarf round my neck to make everybody wonder whether I'd got a sore throat. Friends seeing me wearing a scarf had been known to offer me lozenges.

I was also to envy Mrs Beauchamp her knack of wearing jewellery. She had a weakness for large and flashy adornments, none of which by some miracle ever looked flashy on her. Baubles as big as pigeon eggs hung down from her ears and beads as big as marbles filled the hollow in her neck. Bracelets loaded with charms crashed and jangled at the slightest movement of her delicate wrists and rings dazzled the eye whenever she lifted a finger. I was never sure whether any of the gems were genuine but it didn't seem to matter. Without them Mrs Beauchamp would have felt undressed.

After a few words of welcome I took them to the tiny flatlet and left them no doubt wondering how they were going to fit the van load of furniture that had just arrived into the limited space available. I had other things to think about. I wondered how somebody like Mrs Beauchamp would fit in with her less blue-blooded neighbours and how she would react when Mrs Marsh stood on her step asking for the loan of a bit of sugar. I hoped she wouldn't be too put out.

When I went across later to see how the new arrival had settled in her son had gone. She beamed when she saw me and invited me in. The room, though somewhat overcrowded, already had a comfortable, lived-in look. There were small pieces of furniture strategically placed, china on the built-in dresser, bric-a-brac on the mantelpiece, and on a chair by the fire sat Mrs Marsh. She jumped out of it hurriedly when she saw me.

'It's all right, I'm just on me way,' she said guiltily, holding up an empty cup. 'I only dropped in to see if the lady happened to have a grain of sugar she could lend me until tomorrow. I could have sworn I'd got some in the cupboard but when I looked there was no more than you could lay on a sixpence.' She handed the cup to Mrs Beauchamp who filled it and handed it back. From the things on the table it was clear that Mrs Marsh had already had her first cup of tea with Mrs Beauchamp. It was to be the first of many.

'There you are, my dear,' said Mrs Beauchamp steering her through the door. 'If there's anything else you need don't hesitate to come and ask.'

'Ta muchly, mate, see you later then, if we're not all dead by then,' said Mrs Marsh.

'I'm so sorry about that,' I said, after the door had slammed. 'I hope she wasn't too much of a nuisance. I'm afraid she's got a habit of going round borrowing cups of sugar when she's feeling lonely and wants someone to talk to.'

'Of course she wasn't a nuisance,' said Mrs Beauchamp happily. 'I enjoyed having her. She reminded me terribly of a servant we used to have at the Manor when I was a child. She always wore shoes with the toes and sides cut out. She had dreadful trouble with her feet, poor dear. But of course it couldn't have been her, could it? Sarah could only have been in her forties and Mrs Marsh is getting on, isn't she?' I thought of my mother again. She had got into a chronological muddle towards the end of her life.

But in spite of the muddle and the little mental lapses which Mrs Beauchamp frequently had, it seemed that Mrs Marsh had at last found a friend; a friend she could turn to not only when she ran out of sugar but when she wanted a different fireside to sit beside and someone to talk to. I was as pleased as they were at the way things had gone.

Mrs Beauchamp was full of surprises. One minute she would be holding court, bracelets jangling and rings flashing, while she recalled episodes in her past which she vividly remembered, the next she was wandering through the grounds in search of the gardener, not the Lodge gardener but the gardener of her childhood, and of her girlhood, and of the early days of her married life. When she found the Lodge gardener, usually down on his rheumaticky knees pricking out his seedlings, she would give him a list of vegetables she wanted brought in for the dinner party she was giving that night, and tell him what flowers she would need. And he, recognizing a lady when he saw one in spite of her little lapses, would touch his cap and listen respectfully, then walk her back to her flat and wait until the kettle boiled. He didn't mind at all being mistaken for somebody long since dead.

Every morning soon after nine o'clock she pulled on one of her woolly caps, threw a scarf nonchalantly round her neck and set off for the shops. And at ten she was back. It was then that I arranged the round so that I would be on her doorstep soon after she had unpacked the shopping basket. I knew there would be coffee (not instant) waiting for me, and crusty bread still warm from the baker's oven. While I drank the coffee and tried to resist the temptation to eat too much of the delicious bread, Mrs Beauchamp would tell me things about herself which explained why she was living next door to Mrs Marsh instead of being the mistress of a vast house, waited on hand and foot by servants, as she had once been.

Her fortunes, it seemed, had taken a turn for the worse after she had married a man who was something important in a distant part of the British Empire. 'We had a great many servants in those days,' she said, absentmindedly buttering a tea plate and passing it to me. 'They were all black, of course, but that didn't matter nearly as much then as it does today. They knew they were black and they knew they were servants. None of them would have expected to be treated like ordinary people.' By 'ordinary people' I rightly supposed that she meant the lucky ones who were white and belonged to the ruling classes like her and her husband. 'Such a pity that things have gone the way they have. With all this talk of equality nobody knows their place any longer, and nobody seems to have any respect for their betters. What do you think about it all, my dear?' I hadn't given the matter much thought. Though I was white I definitely didn't belong to the ruling classes and I had been taught by my mother to respect my betters and had gone on doing so right through my training days and far beyond. I had never had any difficulty in knowing who they were. I knew nothing about servants, black or white, so I was in no position to comment on the changes that time had brought to the domestic scene. And even if I had been unwise enough to comment, I might have come down heavily on the side of those who served, rather than upholding the principle of the opposing side. My mother had been a True Blue Tory, but that had never deterred her from being a shareholder in the Co-operative Society. I was as mixed about where I belonged as she was.

If Mrs Beauchamp was going over her past history while she was having one of her little lapses things could get very confusing. One of the particularly puzzling accounts she gave me was of the picnics she and her husband used to have in the copper belt. It was made more confusing by my rather limited grasp of geography. If anybody had asked me where the copper belt was I should have had to admit I didn't know. When I heard about journeys there with a handful of servants and apples I wasn't as impressed as I should have been. With all the money Mr and Mrs B must have had, I would have expected the servants to go staggering through the swamps or the jungle, or whatever led to the copper belt, with great hampers full of exciting things to eat. Apples seemed to be a poor substitute for the wild strawberries and caviar which I had read in romantic novels were the staple diet of the rich. But as I had read the romances when I was very young I could only assume that times had changed since then.

'Were you terribly fond of apples?' I asked Mrs Beauchamp one day after I had listened yet again to a description of the picnics.

'We absolutely adored apples,' she said, her eyes lighting up as if she was savouring the crunchiness of a Cox's Pippin at that very moment.

'But didn't you take other things to eat?' I asked, still thinking that I would have needed something more sustaining after the long trek into the copper belt. I had already gathered that it took several hours to get to the picnic area.

'Other things to eat than what?' asked Mrs Beauchamp, staring at me in puzzlement.

'Other things to eat than apples,' I answered. A look of acute distress came over her face. For a moment I thought she was about to have one of her lapses but on a larger scale.

'But you surely don't imagine that we ate our beautiful apples?' She put her coffee cup down on the table. 'Whatever made you think such a terrible thing?'

'Then what did you do with them when you took them with you on the picnics?' By now I was thoroughly mystified.

'Apples wasn't a them, he was a beautiful Siamese cat. We took him with us wherever we went in those happier times. How could you have possibly thought we would eat him? We were not cannibals you know, even if we did live close to the jungle.' I chose that moment to have one of my more spectacular hot flushes and escaped from the room in search of fresh air. She was still puzzling over my stupidity when I did the round the next day. She gave me some very funny looks while she was pouring out the coffee.

It was some time later that I heard the story of the faithless Mr Beauchamp. Until I did I had visions of him in a pith helmet and rather long shorts, being eaten by something ferocious that had beaten him to the kill. I was wrong again. The truth was less gory but more romantic. Mrs Marsh and I sat enthralled while Mrs Beauchamp unfolded the story.

In spite of the fond memories she had of her husband it seemed that he had gone out of her life when their son was still a little boy. He was but a shadowy figure in his biographer's mind.

'Was he, er, killed, or did he die a natural death?' I asked, egged on by Mrs Marsh, who was sitting in her favourite chair by the fire. She had long since stopped using a shortage of sugar as an excuse to visit her neighbour. She didn't even have to knock before she entered. The friendship between the two women of such different backgrounds had ripened rapidly. Each tolerated the other's little eccentricities and neither of them was in the least concerned about class distinction.

'Was who killed?' asked Mrs Beauchamp, who quickly lost the thread of a conversation and whose memory of immediate things shortened as her memory of the past grew longer. Mrs Marsh raised her eyes to heaven. She hadn't lost her memory at all and sometimes found it hard to be patient with her friend when she strayed from the matter in hand.

'We're talking about your old man,' she said irritably.

'The matron was asking you whether he died in bed natural like or whether he got clobbered by one of them servants you keep telling us about.'

'Or was he savaged by a wild animal?' I breathed. Mrs Beauchamp examined one of her rings and giggled. She had a very girlish giggle.

'It was nothing like that at all,' she said, buffing the ring on the sleeve of her jumper. 'He ran off with Florence and as far as I know they are both still very much alive.'

'And who might Florence be when she's at home?' asked Mrs Marsh, sparing me the indignity of having to ask. Though it was part of my duties to listen sympathetically to things that were told me I made it a rule never to press too hard for further information, however curious I had become. Mrs Beauchamp spread her fingers and breathed on another ring.

'Florence was the young woman we had sent from England to be our darling Evelyn's governess.'

'You never mentioned to me that you'd got a daughter,' said Mrs Marsh.

'I haven't got a daughter,' replied Mrs Beauchamp, obviously wondering how such a mistaken idea could have arisen.

'Then who was your darling Evelyn?' asked Mrs Marsh, determined to get the cast right before we all got too bogged down with the scenario.

'Darling Evelyn is my son,' said Mrs Beauchamp quite unaware of the bomb she had dropped.

'Gawd,' exclaimed Mrs Marsh after she had recovered a little from the shock. 'What a name to give a boy.' She sniggered. 'I bet he didn't half get his leg pulled at school.'

While Mrs Beauchamp was trying to work out why her son should have got his leg pulled at the frightfully expensive school he went to, I explained in an undertone to Mrs Marsh that the name Evelyn could belong either to a girl or boy, adding that it was usually only the upper classes who bestowed it on their sons.

'A bloody good job an' all,' she said. 'He'd have got more than his leg pulled if he'd turned up to work at the Market with a name like that.' She went on to tell me about one or two of the ceremonies performed by the humpers to initiate apprentices. They would certainly have given Evelyn a bad time.

Mrs Beauchamp began to speak and I shut Mrs Marsh up and sat back to listen.

'It all happened in the most curious way,' she said. 'When the young woman arrived he took one look at her and was besotted. They went off together soon after that. It quite ruined his career, of course, which I thought was terribly sad.'

'Sad my eye,' said Mrs Marsh. 'He deserved all he

got. And I suppose you just let him go and didn't so much as lift a finger to get him back.'

'I wouldn't have dreamed of trying to get him back,' said Mrs Beauchamp sharply, looking suddenly like the very proud lady she had always been. 'It wasn't considered ladylike in those days to parade one's feelings in public. It was very different then than it is now when even the best people allow their private lives to be written about in the papers. So undignified I always think. And besides, there was poor Florence to be thought of. Such a pity she was one of the lower classes. It can't have been easy for her suddenly finding herself in a position so far above her station. No, I simply brought Apples and Evelyn home when everything had been settled.'

'More fool you,' said Mrs Marsh. 'I'd have given them both a bloody good hiding if I'd been in your shoes.' Mrs Beauchamp thought hard for a moment then turned a puzzled face to her friend.

'But why should I have given them the sort of good hiding you mentioned? Darling Evelyn was only a little boy and poor dear Apples was already going blind in one eye. Neither of them was in any way responsible for my troubles.'

'Oh, my good Gawd,' groaned Mrs Marsh. 'She's off again. The poor old cow gets barmier every day.' I left them sorting out the confusion between Mr Beauchamp, Florence, Apples and darling Evelyn. I knew from experience that it would take time.

But despite the little lapses, and the different wavelengths they were all too frequently on, the two old ladies were almost as close as sisters. Even closer than some. It wasn't long before Mrs Marsh was setting out to buy her jellied eels wearing a pair of egg-sized earrings that brushed the collar of her old tweed coat. Occasionally there was the clank of a charm-loaded bracelet as she lifted her work-worn hand, and eventually the old tweed coat was replaced by an old fur coat that smelled strongly of mothballs. But nothing replaced the slashed up shoes. Her friend's feet were several sizes smaller than hers.

There was only one fly in the ointment to mar Mrs Marsh's enjoyment of the fineries she was either lent or given. 'It's a pity there isn't a pop shop anywhere handy,' she said wistfully one day. 'Some of them bracelets and things she lends me would fetch a bob or two to tide me over when I get short before me pension's due.' I was glad there wasn't a pop shop handy. I had enough to do without having to rush to a pawn shop to get Mrs Marsh out of trouble. I had already caught her once trying to palm the fur coat off onto a tally man in payment for a pair of sheets she'd had on tick.

Mrs Beauchamp's life took an entirely new turn after Mrs Marsh introduced her to bingo. For a long time she had been under the impression that Bingo was the name of an old and faithful dog which her friend visited every Wednesday afternoon at some nearby kennels called the Hall. She said that she would be delighted to meet Bingo. She remembered one of the under-gardeners at the Manor having a dog called Bingo but she was never allowed to touch him. Nanny always said he might bite.

Mrs Marsh had been playing bingo every Wednesday for a long time. The hall where she played had once been a cinema. It was where I was sitting one afternoon at the beginning of the war when the manager came and told us that there was a bomb in an apple tree at the sanatorium on top of the hill. The announcement had brought the film to a halt and changed a great many people's lives.

Mrs Marsh's addiction to bingo hadn't brought her to ruin; neither did it make her rich. The most she ever won at a session was barely enough to cover the cost of a cup of tea and a biscuit – or a packet of crisps – in the interval before the next session. On the many occasions when she hadn't won anything at all she came home raging at the disparity in the distribution of wealth which allowed one to emerge from the bingo hall with a bulging purse and another with next to nothing. Mrs Marsh had never had a bulging purse. And even if she had suddenly acquired one it wouldn't have stayed bulging for long. She lived for the day, knowing that with a bit of luck somebody would take care of tomorrow.

After one or two of the more difficult rules about playing bingo had been explained over and over again as simply as possible and Mrs Beauchamp appeared to have grasped them, the two friends set out together one Wednesday afternoon. Mrs Beauchamp had been in a state of excitement all morning. She was always willing to experiment with something new and had even started to acquire a taste for jellied eels. It hadn't been easy. Once, when her friend was out of earshot she confided in me that in her opinion the eels were overrated. They were not nearly as delicious as oysters and she had had great trouble with the tiny bones when she had tried to swallow them whole. Having eaten neither an eel nor an oyster I was in no position to make comparisons. But I agreed with her comments on eels as I would have agreed with Mrs Marsh's comments on oysters.

The first bingo outing was a great success. I went across specially that evening to hear all about it. Contrary to Mrs Marsh's gloomy predictions that her friend would as likely as not have one of her little lapses just as the winning number was being called, it had gone off without a hitch. Apart from asking what the caller meant when he said Kelly's eye and clickety-click, she had required no help at all from anybody. Mrs Marsh was very proud of her.

'Caught on quick, she did,' she said, looking fondly down at her apt pupil. 'She'd properly got the hang of it when we started the second game. And considering that it was the first time she'd played, and how daft she is sometimes, it was bloody marvellous the way she picked it up.' Mrs Beauchamp graciously accepted the back-handed compliment then hastened to correct its inaccuracies.

'But it isn't the first time I've played,' she said. 'I played it often with Nanny and sometimes even with dear Papa. But it was called Lotto then and, of course, we didn't play for money. Papa would never have allowed that. He didn't approve of gambling.' Mrs Marsh muttered something rude about Papa and I left them holding an inquest on the afternoon's play.

Chapter Six

NOT ONLY WAS the Lodge lacking in the up-to-date amenities which the modern glossy homes provided for their residents, it lacked other things that would have made life easier for us all.

Over the years the original gas light-fittings had been ruthlessly torn out and electricity installed; a cooker was put in every flat, making the old-fashioned range necessary only for raising the temperature to a degree which I found unbearable; and the copper in the corner of the kitchen had been dealt with as ruthlessly as the gas light-fittings.

The innovations hadn't been welcomed by everybody. I heard stories of former residents who had preferred to sit in the dark rather than tamper with switches they didn't understand; and those who had cooked on an all-purpose range since the day they got married didn't take kindly to the new-fangled thing in the kitchen. Losing the copper was perhaps the unkindest cut of all. Wash day was never the same without it. Whites lost their whiteness through not being boiled and no amount of scrubbing restored their snowy appearance. After living for more than seventy years doing things one way it wasn't easy to have to start doing them another.

But one thing remained as it had been since the Lodge was built. Tucked down at one end between the place where the odd job man kept his tools and the place where everything got stored when there was no immediate use for it was the bathroom. It was very basic, and largely unused.

When the plans were drawn up by the charitable body of the day nobody had given much thought to luxuries like bathrooms. The custom of regular bathing hadn't spread to the lower classes. It was only the rich who considered it essential to have a daily immersion in water. It wasn't surprising therefore that one bathroom had been thought enough to satisfy the needs of twenty ladies, especially as the twenty were all of reduced circumstances and presumably not accustomed to taking baths, or certainly not since they had become needy enough to qualify for one of the flatlets.

The bathroom was small, cold and comfortless. It contained a very large bath, which stood on four iron feet and had a long streak of brown staining running from the cold tap. Apart from cobwebs, the only other thing in the bathroom was a slatted wooden board for stepping out onto.

'When do you have a bath?' I asked Mrs Turgoose after I had been at the Lodge long enough to notice that there were no queues outside the door of the nasty little room, and no ladies in bathrobes wandering along the verandah on Saturday nights or any other nights. Mrs Turgoose bridled.

'I hope you're not suggesting that I don't look after meself properly,' she said crossly. I assured her that I wasn't suggesting anything of the sort, I was merely wondering why nobody seemed to use the bathroom.

'There was a woman once who used to use it,' said Mrs Turgoose, 'but that was only because she was a bit stuck up and tried to make out she was better than us. She soon went off the idea when it started to get cold.'

'Wouldn't you like to have a bath?' I said to Mrs Marsh one day when I caught her having a good wash down in front of her fire.

'Not me,' she said. 'I catch cold quick enough without sitting about in water up to my neck. Personally I don't believe in it. You can keep yourself clean without all that palaver.'

When I mentioned to Mrs Beauchamp about having

a bath she said she had one every Sunday when she went to her son's for lunch. She had begged Mrs Marsh to go with her but Mrs Marsh had raised every obstacle.

'What if that lad of yours was to walk in when I was in the middle of it?' she said.

'But of course he wouldn't, dear,' said Mrs Beauchamp. 'The door would be locked so that nobody could get in.'

'And what if I was to pass away suddenly and they had to break the door down to get at me? Besides, I don't fancy the idea of a lot of men breaking the door down and me without a stitch on.' Nothing Mrs Beauchamp said would persuade her friend to accept the invitation to go and have a bath.

Even after improvements were made and a fan heater was put in there was still only a trickle of ladies venturing out on Saturday nights on their way to the bathroom. There were never enough to make it necessary to draw up a roster.

As well as the prehistoric bathroom there were other signs that the Lodge had been built a long time ago and hadn't kept up with the changing times. It had originally been intended to give shelter to twenty ladies who were of good character and in reasonably good health. There was a matron in residence and on call for twenty-four hours a day. Her duties in the main were to make sure that nobody looked ill, felt ill, or was ill without proper steps being taken to deal with the crisis before it got out of hand. It was easier in those days to take the proper steps.

If the complaint was only trifling the doctor was sent for and the patient assured in a good, old-fashioned bedside manner that all would be well if she took the little pills he gave her. And it usually was.

If the complaint was rather more serious, the doctor was sent for and the nearest female relatives asked to come in several times a day bringing nourishing slops and plenty of clean linen and nightdresses. If necessary they would be instructed to take it in turns to sit up at night with Auntie, Granny or Mother. Nobody minded any of this; they saw it as their duty.

But if things got worse and the little pills and nourishing slops weren't enough, there was always a bed in the infirmary ready and waiting, however reluctant the patient was to go.

Things were different when I got to the Lodge. Doctors were too busy to do house visits when it seemed that all that was needed was a prescription which could be collected from the surgery. Daughters and other female relatives were too busy going out to work to make nourishing slops, and too tired when the day was over to keep an all-night vigil at a bedside; and hospitals were too busy to have beds ready and waiting for an old lady whose only claim to one might be that she was dying.

The result of the changes that had come about in recent years meant that more of the responsibility for caring for the residents had fallen on the matron and whatever help she could get from the Social Services. Home-helps were applied for and meals-on-wheels ordered. But at the weekends and on all other days when the home-helps stayed at home and the meals-on-wheels didn't come, it was often the matron who had to cook dainty little invalid meals, and it was often the matron who had to go out and shop for the ingredients.

It was too often the matron who sat for long hours in the night listening to the rattle of labouring lungs, and praying that the doctor who was new to the neighbourhood would get there in time, and if he did that he would ring the hospital and ask for a bed, and that there would be a bed available.

I had been working at the Lodge for more than a year before it was decided that there was enough money in the charitable kitty to employ another pair of hands to enable me to have one day off a week and a free weekend each month. Until then I was on call twenty-four hours a day for seven days a week. This kept me very busy, especially when Miss May took to her bed as she often did.

Miss May was tall and angular. She had high and prominent cheek bones which were flushed with feverish pink. Her myopic eyes stared out from gold-rimmed spectacles and her black hair, without a silver thread among it, was coiled round her head in several wispy plaits. She had proudly told me once that she had enjoyed ill health since the midwife wrapped her in a shawl, made the sign of a cross on her little wizened brow and informed everybody that the poor wee mite wouldn't live long enough to be properly baptized. The poor wee mite had surprised them all. She had been wearing shawls for eighty years when I first met her and was busily crocheting another to wear on her next birthday.

I liked Miss May. Everybody liked her. And because she was so well liked, and because of the frail look and the flushed cheeks she only had to hint that she wanted a little job done to get it done at once. The vicar, who dropped in twice a week to pray for her soul, found himself doing the most unexpected things. The doctor, who firmly believed that she was well enough to rise from her bed and walk to the lavatory instead of ringing her bell for me to put her on the commode, was amazed when he heard himself telling her that she was quite right in thinking that she should stay in bed for at least another week. He also walked to his car wondering what spell she had put on him to persuade him to fill the coal scuttle and make a small adjustment to a drooping curtain before he left. He had been her doctor long enough to know that neither he nor anybody else was allowed to leave Miss May's flat before they had done some small thing to improve her lot. Her lot was a very happy one in spite of the ill-health that she declared had dogged her from the cradle.

I was no more impervious to her spells than the vicar or the doctor. Whenever a bell rang out not ten minutes after I had finished a round I knew without looking at the indicator board who would be ringing. That I had only so recently left Miss May as well as could be expected was no guarantee that she wouldn't have found a dozen reasons for wanting me back. The reasons were often feeble: there was a speck of dust on the dresser that the home-help, who had just left, had overlooked; there was an ornament on the mantelpiece an inch off centre; or there was a faint smell of something which Miss May was convinced was gas escaping from a fractured pipe; or a tap that hadn't been properly turned off. She was very nervous about gas. She was already at the Lodge when the cookers were first put in. She had written long and involved letters to the committee explaining that she was of a nervous disposition and feared that something awful would happen to her if she meddled with the new contraption. They sent a man to show her how to turn on the tap and apply a match but she was a slow learner. Even after I got there she still lacked confidence. She would turn on a tap, strike a match, then back away in terror before the gas ignited. It was then that she rang her bell for me to go and save her from asphyxiation.

She was nervous about other things as well. When a little Russian dog was sent to the moon she sat at her window dreading the moment when it would miss its footing and come hurtling from the skies and onto one of our lawns. Later, when man followed dog she trembled to think of the damage a hefty man dressed in a space suit could do to her roof if he fell over the side of the moon. 'But surely,' she said, 'those who planned the project would have foreseen the dangers and forestalled them?' I assured her they would.

Miss May was always grateful for the things that were done for her. She would take whoever's hand had done them in her fleshless fingers, plant a kiss in the palm and, her eyes brimming with tears, would beg their pardon for being such a nuisance and sob that it would be a blessing for all when she was gone. When she had been passionately assured that nothing was further from the truth, she would dry her eyes and immediately think up something else she wanted done.

But of all the things that were done out of love or duty for Miss May when she came over queer, preparing her meals was the most exhausting. Somewhere around the time when she was crocheting her fiftieth shawl her doctor had warned her, yet again, that her days were numbered. He had suggested that in order to prolong them she should eat small meals at frequent intervals. This she did, by day and night, gaining not an ounce in the next thirty years.

The first experience I had of Miss May's regular eating times came shortly after I started at the Lodge. I was wakened in the middle of the night by her emergency bell and raced down the garden path, certain that I would find her breathing her last. I slackened my pace when I realized that if she were indeed *in extremis* she wouldn't have had the strength to get out of bed and ring the bell.

Positioning the bells when they were first put in had given the planners quite a few headaches. Given that almost as many elderly people become suddenly ill while sitting comfortably by the fireside as are stricken when they are lying in bed, short of having emergency bells all over the place there can be no guarantee that one will be at hand when needed. With this in mind the bells in the flats were placed midway between bed and fire, thus ensuring that they would be equally inaccessible from either side.

Miss May wasn't *in extremis*. She was in bed, weary with journeying to and from her bell. She apologized tearfully for fetching me out but explained that it was two o'clock and time for her Milo, and since she had come over queer and couldn't get it herself, she had had no option but to ring for me. She rang for me again at five; and again at eight; and at three-hourly intervals throughout the day. On the numerous occasions that Miss May came over queer and took to her bed I went wearily to mine, praying that the little snack I had given her at midnight might just for once keep her finger off the bell until cornflake time came round again.

Once, in a moment of desperation brought on by fatigue, I had tentatively suggested that maybe the meals-on-wheels ladies would fill the one o'clock void from Monday to Friday. The suggestion hadn't been well received. Miss May had seized my hand in hers, planted on it so many kisses and wept so many tears of remorse that, after I had finished telling her that she wasn't a nuisance and mustn't think of dying, I vowed that only over my own dead body would a meal on a wheel be allowed to cross the threshold. I went on grilling and braising, toasting and poaching exactly as if the ladies of the WRVS had never existed.

At first, when Miss May came to live at the Lodge, a veritable army of helpers had beaten a path to her front door. Ministers, vicars, priests and pastors had vied with each other to guide her faltering footsteps towards the promised land. Friends and neighbours and a saintly distant cousin called Sid had rallied round to give the help they were so often called upon to give. While one swept, another dusted, and others rolled up their sleeves and scrubbed and polished. Some brought piles of clean washing in discreetly covered baskets, and some arrived with dainty little dishes which only needed to be popped in the oven when required. One of the ministers who was good at woodwork kept the chair legs from falling off and a Roman Catholic priest, who by rights shouldn't have been there at all, painted the doors in a sensible, labour-saving mahogany colour. There was a young man on the premises who was paid a modest wage for mending chair legs and painting woodwork but Miss May said she didn't like to trouble him. What were friends for if they couldn't be relied on to do the occasional little odd job?

But gradually through natural causes and for various reasons the army of helpers dwindled. Soon all that was left of the old brigade was the wife of the minister who was good at sticking back chair legs, and the saintly Sid. He was the last to go.

I heard about Sid while I was working my way through a list of little tasks which Miss May had jotted down so that I wouldn't forget them. She was in bed at the time, having a few days' rest to recover from the few days when she had felt well enough to get up. The reason I was doing the little tasks was because the home-help who should have been doing them had rung to say her daughter was having a baby and she wouldn't be back until it was all over. I could only hope that it would all be over quickly. The chances of getting another home-help were very remote; they were in short supply.

Twice a week for years Sid had boarded a succession of buses, not all of them immediately connecting, and had crossed many acres of suburbia to get to his ailing cousin. He had come with plenty of protective clothing to save his best suit from getting ruined while he was tidying up the coal cellar, thrusting a brush up the chimney to dislodge a bird's nest or loosen some impacted soot, and climbing on ladders to clean the outside windows. Hardly stopping to snatch a bite of the dinner he cooked for his cousin, Sid had slaved from the moment he got there to the moment he left.

On the remaining days of the week, except for Sunday, he had boarded other buses and travelled in different directions to perform similar acts of kindness for other distant cousins. He had truly earned the eternal rest he was called to suddenly while he was sitting on a bus with his protective clothing tied up in a bundle.

'It couldn't have happened at a worse time,' said Miss May mournfully, dabbing her eyes at the memory. 'I'd just been under the doctor and he'd warned me that if I carried on the way I was doing he couldn't promise anything. I was relying on Sid to come and change the bed just in case. But instead of turning up on Tuesday as he always did he went off to somebody's funeral, caught his death and went the following Friday on his way over here. I never thought Sid would have left me like that.'

I plumped up her pillows, gave her a sip of lemon and barley water and said how sorry I was to hear of the tragedy that had befallen her cousin. And so I was. Men like Sid are hard to find, and are not easily replaced when they go. He must have been as sadly missed by the other distant cousins as he was by Miss May.

Chapter Seven

As well as having to learn as quickly as possible which were the extroverts among the residents and which were of a less gregarious nature, it was necessary for me to distinguish between the thrifty and those who foolishly clung to the idea that money was for spending, however little of it there might be. Mrs Marsh, who had always lived beyond her income and was still happily squandering her old age pension on bingo and jellied eels, looked down her nose at Mrs Drew who had never spent sixpence without first making sure that she was getting value for every penny. And Mrs Turgoose, whose idea of heaven was a drop of gin and a sing-song, thought very poorly of little Miss Coombe who kept herself to herself in the corner and never touched a drop except for a small glass of sherry at Christmas.

The more I considered the alternative ways of growing old the more confused I was about which to choose for myself. Sometimes it seemed that it would be more fun to be like Mrs Marsh and let the pension money – when I became eligible for it – slip through my fingers like water, splashing out on liver and onions one day with scarcely enough for an eel the next. Then I remembered her old tweed coat which she had worn for so long before she exchanged it for Mrs Beauchamp's old musquash, and wondered whether it wouldn't perhaps be wiser to follow Mrs Drew's example.

Mrs Drew had been thrifty all her life, saving with almost religious fervour for the rainy day which never came. The money that had accumulated would never bring her happiness. She would continue to eat her frugal meals, and wear the same shiny, well-preserved serge coat and skirt she told me she had worn since before the war. Which war she was talking about I wasn't sure, but from the cut and style, and the quality of the material, it could have been the Great War! Any suggestion that she should treat herself to a new dress, or buy a more modern wireless set to replace the one that crackled and spat when she turned it on, was received with shock.

'And just where do you think the money's going to come from for such extravagances?' she wanted to know. It was no business of mine to tell her, or even to hint that it could have come from the rainy-day savings. She wouldn't have listened anyway. Thinking about the money lying safely in the bank gave her a feeling of security which no amount of pretty dresses or new wireless sets could ever have done. She had known so much hardship in her life that she had vowed long ago never to be penniless again, once things started to improve, even if it meant going without the things she could afford to buy. The vow had kept her putting patches on her pinnies until she was patching patches, and making do with minuscule amounts of mince when she could have afforded a bit of best rump.

The first time she asked me to go out and buy the mince I went willingly, though with some misgivings. I knew she would never have asked if she could have gone herself, but after she fell and broke a leg she had to rely on others to do her shopping. She wasn't always happy with the things they bought. Or with the price they had paid.

'How much shall I bring?' I asked. She wrinkled her brow and chewed the end of the pencil she was using to work out the cost of the mince.

'I suppose it will have to be a quarter of a pound,' she said at last. 'What with the gristle and the fat there'll be nothing left of it by the time it's cooked. And furthermore, I'd rather you got it from that butcher at the far end of the town. I don't trust the one round the corner. He's short-changed me more than once.'

The butcher at the far end of the town weighed the mince with precision, adding and subtracting a morsel or two until the hands of the scales registered exactly four ounces.

'You'll be the new matron at the Lodge I shouldn't wonder,' he said, pushing his straw hat to the back of his head. 'You'd better have a receipt for this little lot. It's for Mrs Drew no doubt and she likes to know how her money's being spent.'

Mrs Drew took the tiny package from me, carefully counted the change, noted that there was a halfpenny less than she had expected and weighed the mince. Only when she had satisfied herself that there wasn't a grain short did she grudgingly thank me for running the errand. I was grateful to the butcher for giving me a receipt. Without it I would have had to do a lot of explaining about the halfpenny deficit.

The broken leg took a long time to mend. It was a great trial to Mrs Drew, who valued her independence. But with the aid of two sticks and a tea trolley she managed in a way that astonished me. Unlike Miss May, who, as Miss Nightingale was said to have done when her mission was completed, lay back on her virgin couch directing operations, she did all she could for herself.

When they sent Mrs Drew from the hospital with her leg in plaster she took the chewed-up pencil and planned a timetable. The tea trolley was an indispensable part of the plan. It became walking aid, mobile kitchen and bathroom. Supported by its sturdy frame she hobbled round her flat. Sitting in a chair beside it she peeled her potatoes, washed her cabbage and prepared whatever else she was having for lunch. Or she propped herself up by it while she cut bread and butter, put saucepans on the cooker and things in the oven. And when the meal was ready she laid a lacy little cloth on the top tier and ate in style.

Morning and evening she used the trolley as a bathroom, putting soap and flannel, towels and talcum powder and a plentiful supply of hot water on each of the tiers. Not once did Mrs Drew ring her bell and ask me to make her a nice cup of tea or give her a blanket bath.

She kept strictly to the timetable. By noon she was ready to sit down for lunch and when the dishes were done she composed herself for her afternoon nap. At two she was awake and ready to receive visitors. She had her tea at four and was starting to get ready for bed by six o'clock. Anybody rash enough to knock at her door between one and two or after six found her not at home to callers.

Even the baker arranged his round to be at her door when her afternoon nap was over. Her life was so organized that any deviation from normal routine threw her off balance, and put her into a very bad temper.

'If you can't come at a respectable time I'd rather you didn't come at all,' she told those who arrived out of hours, often shouting the injunction through the letter box.

Mrs Drew didn't like home-helps. She made things hard for them. Consequently they came and went, leaving me to cope in their absence with the assistance of a kind lady from one of the churches. The lady was very patient. She knew exactly how to handle difficult people like Mrs Drew. She never said an argumentative word, never rubbed them up the wrong way and never looked in the least bit pained however much they stormed. I, alas, did all these things. I was often tempted to snap when Mrs Drew insisted that I hadn't done something when I knew I had, and I got quite argumentative when the change I brought back from the shopping was counted over and over again to prove that her calculations were right and mine wrong. I looked extremely pained when the decimal coins were confused with the old-fashioned sort, though I was almost as much confused about those as she was. It took me a long time to understand how a shilling could have been reduced to fivepence overnight and how a two shilling piece should be worth only tenpence.

But despite the number of times that we failed to see eye to eye, Mrs Drew gradually began to trust me enough to ask me in when I did a round. Occasionally she mentioned that she wasn't expecting callers that afternoon, and if I had time she would be only too pleased if I went and had a chat. She had obviously forgiven me for the errors I made when I was totting up the expenditure. She let me sit in one of her creaking basket chairs while she told me things which gave me a better understanding of why she wasn't the easiest woman to get on with.

Her mother had been a gentle soul, bullied and beaten by a drunken husband. She had been forced to work far into the night sewing tiny pearls on rich gowns in order that her large brood of children would have enough to eat. Mrs Drew had more than a touch of bitterness in her voice when she told me that as she left childhood behind and saw the way that women were made to suffer she had made up her mind that no man would treat her as her mother was treated. And none ever had.

'But you got married, didn't you?' I said. She looked up from the stocking she was darning.

'Yes, I got married, but I let it be known from the start that I wasn't going to be a doormat for a man to wipe his feet on.' I thought of Mrs Pankhurst who had probably had the same revolutionary ideas which had led to her Suffragette Movement.

'How did you manage to get the message across?' I asked.

Mrs Drew smiled grimly. 'I wore the trousers and I held the purse strings. It's being dependent on what a man cares to give you out of his pay packet that makes a woman feel inferior. I took his pay packet off him the moment he got in on Friday night, gave him his pocket money and kept the rest for the housekeeping and saved what was left over for a rainy day.' I sat for a moment thinking of my parents.

My mother hadn't exactly worn the trousers but she had held the purse strings. She had given my father half-a-crown a week and had kept the rest of his wages, using what she needed for the housekeeping and depositing the remainder in the Co-op bank.

It had stayed there accumulating interest, until one day after my father died, and while she was still in a state of shock, she had gone to the bank and drawn all of it out. Then she had carefully wrapped the notes, of which there were many, in paper doilies and used them to light the fire.

Remembering this I couldn't help thinking that maybe Mrs Drew should have used a little of her money before the habit of saving was impossible to break, and before it was too late to get any enjoyment from it. Though for all I knew my mother might have thoroughly enjoyed lighting her fire with the five pound notes. She had forgotten all about it when I asked her.

Mrs Drew sat with a faint look of sadness in her eyes. Then, just when I thought it was time for me to be on my way she started to speak again.

'But he wasn't a bad husband as husbands go. He was good about the house and never went out without me. He was a street lamplighter when were first married. I used to follow him round on my bike when he went off in the evening to light the lamps.'

'Whatever for?' I asked, finding it hard to imagine her as a young woman with her skirts hitched up pedalling down the gas-lit streets in the wake of her lamplighter husband.

Again she smiled grimly. 'He was good looking when he was young and if I hadn't kept an eye on him he'd have had all the girls in the town chasing after him.' I could see that as well as wearing the trousers and holding the purse strings she had loved her husband with a jealous possessiveness.

I had to wait for a while before Mrs Drew told me something which none of the rumours that buzzed round the Lodge had hinted at. Either it had all happened too long ago for anybody to remember or everybody had lost interest after the nine days of wonder had died down.

'When we found we couldn't have any children we adopted a boy,' she said one afternoon when I was sitting in the creaking basket chair. She was turning a sheet sides to middle. It had been turned so often that it would have been difficult to guess which were the sides and which the middle when it was first bought.

'I didn't know you had a son,' I said.

'I haven't. He ran away from home when he was sixteen. He lied about his age and joined the army. He only came home a time or two after that.' She looked down at the sheet, but not before I had seen a glint of tears.

'Why did he run away?' I asked, then hoped I hadn't gone too far.

'I used to thrash him. If I sent him to the shops and he didn't bring the proper change back I used to let him know that money didn't grow on trees. He seemed to think that it was come by easy and that losing a penny or two didn't matter. But I thrashed him once too often and he ran away.'

'Where is he now?' I asked, knowing that he didn't visit his mother.

'I don't know. The last I heard of him was when his father died. I managed to trace him through the Salvation Army but he didn't come to the funeral. He wrote and said he was married with two children but he never wrote again. He'd never forgiven me for the way I went on at him when he was a lad.' She held the sewing needle up to the light but couldn't thread it. Her eyes were too blurred with tears. I took the needle and cotton off her.

'What did your husband say about it all?' I asked, thinking not for the first time that the little eyes in the needles were getting smaller than they used to be.

'He wasn't one to say much,' she said. 'But I know he missed the boy and he would have liked to have seen the grandchildren. He was fond of children.' I gathered that he had never thrashed his adopted son.

It sounded a sad little story to me, but sad or not, none of what had happened in the past made Mrs Drew any less careful about checking the change when anybody did the shopping for her. Though she couldn't thrash them she had ways of letting them know that money didn't grow on trees. When everybody started talking about 'peas' instead of pence Mrs Drew dropped every half pea into an old cracked cup and unloaded them onto the baker when the cup was full.

Sadly it was the kind old baker who caused Mrs Drew's undoing. Twice a week for years, except for the time when she was in hospital with the broken leg, he had knocked on her door to deliver the small brown Hovis and the three currant buns which she always had. He stood and waited patiently while she, alert after her afternoon nap, trundled her trolley to the door.

On the day that he came a few minutes early Mrs Drew got up from her chair, still half-dazed with sleep, slipped, and added a broken hip to her other infirmities. The two sticks and the tea trolley were no longer of any use.

She never came back to the Lodge and I missed her very much. Later, when I was listening to the nice young parson at the crematorium trying to say kind things about a woman he had never known, I thought about the boy she had adopted. I wished he hadn't been quite so unforgiving. His children might have been a joy to their grandma in her old age and she could have left them her money instead of it all going to a charity. There was enough to buy dozens of new pinnies and a great many more things besides. The rainy day she had so carefully saved for had never come.

Chapter Eight

THE GINGER CAT that was our only four-footed resident had generously allowed me a short settling-in period before he started to become a thorn in my flesh. Through the shortening summer days, and while the mists and fruitfulness of autumn were upon us, he snoozed beneath the trees, hardly twitching a whisker even when sparrows and pigeons pecked around him. When he wasn't under any of the trees he could often be seen sunning himself in the middle of the forecourt and refusing to move no matter how many cars were honking around him, their drivers trying to park prettily as the notices requested them to do; or he was flattening the perennials in the herbaceous borders which were the pride and joy of our old gardener.

The gardener had been tending the roses and the herbaceous borders since he was a young man. As well as passionately caring for annuals and bi-annuals, he would water all the little pot plants while their owners were away. Busy lizzies burst into bloom at his touch and mother-in-law's tongues seemed all the sharper for his attentions.

His geraniums were a blaze of colour long after less nurtured ones had withered; and his roses were so uncompromisingly pruned at the proper time that they managed to survive the wettest and windiest of flaming Junes and went on blooming until well after the autumn equinox. A few even lasted until Christmas but they were beginning to look a bit bedraggled by then.

Not a single weed popped up without being detected at once and ruthlessly plucked out, and no dandelion puffs defiled the velvety smoothness of the lawns. The gardens were a pleasure to behold; they would have been a pleasure to sit in on warm sunny days if any of the residents had taken advantage of the seats that were scattered around the grounds for just that purpose. But none of them did. They preferred a comfortable chair by the fire to a hard wooden bench surrounded by roses. Only the birds, the pigeons and the ginger cat availed themselves of the peace which the gardens offered, and they sometimes disturbed it with their squabbles over territorial rights.

Though the cat was known by several different names when he was flattening the perennials or clut-

tering up the forecourt, his given name was Tommy.
The story of how he came to live at the Lodge had
touched me deeply when I first heard it. It lost a lot of
its pathos after he and I had become better acquainted.

Tommy belonged to Miss Lilian. She was a spinster
lady, four foot ten and weighing not an ounce over six
and a half stones. Her intellect, which had never been
bright, had grown duller with the onset of age. By the
time she got to the top of the list for one of the flats
she was already having difficulty in knowing what day
of the week it was. She sometimes had trouble in
distinguishing between day and night.

Before her name was put on the list she had kept
house for an old man who, by Miss Lilian's standards,
was very well off. She dreamed dreams of the day he
died and left her all his riches. But, being an avid
reader of the Sunday papers, she knew that even the
most faithful servant was sometimes overlooked when
the wealth was being distributed. With this in mind she
had searched the house from attic to cellar looking for
hiding-places which her miserly employer might have
used to dodge the tax man. When she chanced upon a
few hundred pounds hidden in a dark recess of an
unused chimney she thought about all she'd done for
the old man, and the pittance he paid her and had
decided that none but the most pure in heart would

grudge her the windfall she found up his chimney. She sewed a little pocket in her corsets, stuffed the windfall into it and never breathed a word to a soul.

I came upon the bundle of notes under a pillow one morning when I was making her bed. Usually she was perfectly capable of making her bed herself but she was feeling poorly at the time and though the doctor couldn't make up his mind what was wrong with her, he told her to stay in bed for a day or two and ordered a lot of different things in the hope that if one didn't work another might.

The notes were held together by a sturdy rubber band and were of a larger denomination than any I had seen before. I could feel my eyes widening.

'Whatever's this?' I cried, holding up the bundle. Miss Lilian snatched it off me.

'It's money,' she said.

'I can see it's money, but whose is it and what's it doing under your pillow?' I asked, using the matronly voice I only used under special circumstances. Miss Lilian looked everywhere but at me.

'It's mine and I always keep it under the pillow when I'm not wearing any corsets. When I am I keep it sewn in them.' I went into the kitchen and made her a nice cup of Benger's to loosen her tongue.

She told me about the old man, and how faithfully

she'd served him for longer than she could remember, and the little thanks she'd had for anything she did. Then, rather diffidently, she told me of the search from attic to cellar. When she got to the bit about the chimney I stopped her.

'You shouldn't have kept it,' I told her sternly. 'You should have handed it over to one of the relatives, or taken it round to the old man's solicitor.' Miss Lilian thought about it for a moment.

'If I'd given it to his relations they'd only have spent it, and I've never had any dealings with solicitors.' I decided to let the matter drop. Knowing Miss Lilian and the state her mind got into sometimes she could quite easily have come by the money through the proper channels. And if she hadn't, then it was no part of my duties to sit in judgement on the residents.

Tommy had been Miss Lilian's faithful friend since he was a fluffy kitten. When the old man died and left her homeless, if not quite penniless, she had put her name on the list for a flatlet at the Lodge. In due course she stood before the committee with her faithful friend spitting and snarling in a cat basket. The basket was almost as big as Miss Lilian.

The chairperson had looked askance at the heaving basket then, settling himself in the Chair, had proceeded to read out the rules that had to be obeyed by all who lived at the Lodge. When he got to the one stating that no dog, cat, any other animal, or any feathered friends except a budgerigar, were to be kept on the premises, he looked even more pointedly at the cat basket and gave Miss Lilian the choice between having Tommy put down or forfeiting her right to a flatlet. She unhesitatingly made her choice. She looked round at the ladies and gentlemen sitting at the walnut table and with tears in her eyes she told them that her mind was made up, Tommy would have to go. Whereupon they gave her the key of Flat 4a and wished her a long and happy life in her new home.

It was a week or two after her arrival that she was first seen at the dead of night walking through the grounds with Tommy trailing after her, tied to the end of a long piece of rope. It was another week or two before the committee sent one of their lady members to check on the rumour that Tommy was alive and well and living in Flat 4a. But Miss Lilian had friends, and even before the lady had knocked on her door and been invited in, steps had been taken to make her visit fruitless. She had a quick look under the bed, in the wardrobe, on top of the dresser, and anywhere else where a cat might have been hiding, but without success. She went away convinced that a grave injustice had been done, and at the next committee meeting she as good as told her fellow members that they ought to be ashamed of themselves for thinking ill of such a nice old lady as Miss Lilian. Though some of her fellow members still had doubts, they took her word for it and passed on to more important things.

When Tommy eventually came out of the closet, or wherever he was bundled when there was any danger of him being discovered, he purred so sweetly at those who were again demanding his immediate demise that even the hardest heart was softened and he won a reprieve. Miss Lilian was so happy when she heard the news that she went out at once and bought him a pair of kippers for his tea and a collar with a tiny bell.

It was the ringing of an emergency bell one after-noon that triggered off the first feelings of hatred in my heart for the ginger cat. Bells in the afternoon were not unknown, though it was usually in the middle of the night when they were rung. At first when I went to work at the Lodge my dreams were haunted by peals of imaginary bells. Once, after wakening suddenly from a deep sleep, I grabbed a dressing gown, stum-bled downstairs, banged my head on the banister, ricked my ankle and hobbled to the indicator board, only to realize when I got there that the bell I heard was no more real than Mrs Marsh's Messerschmitts. I went back to bed cold and bruised and just getting drowsy when a real bell rang and off I went again. Being on call for twenty-four hours a day could be very exhausting, especially if there was an epidemic of something racing through the Lodge like a forest fire.

It was Miss Coombe's bell that had shattered the afternoon peace. She was the lady who had taken such interest in the geraniums while Mrs Beauchamp was moving in. She lived in the corner near the bathroom and kept herself so much to herself that some of her neighbours didn't know she was there until she rang her bell.

Her door was open when I got there. She was standing beside a large chromium birdcage weeping bitterly. The cage was empty. Two long green tail feathers lying on the carpet told their own sad story.

Miss Coombe's budgerigar had been a legend in his lifetime. He was large and green, and extremely bad tempered. Nobody ever put a finger between the bars of his cage without wishing they hadn't. His vocabulary was astonishing, his gift for mimicry amazing. 'Good morning, dear, and how are we today?' he simpered sarcastically whenever he saw me. 'Wotcher cock, got a bit of sugar you can lend us?' he called out with heavy humour when, through a chink in the curtains, he spied Mrs Marsh and her empty cup going past the window. He never used swear words. He didn't know any. But a week spent in one of the armed Forces would have given him a repertoire that would have made his mistress blush. There was no doubt that of all the budgerigars that lived in the Lodge he was by far the brightest.

I led the weeping Miss Coombe to a chair and sat down beside her.

'What happened, dear?' I inquired softly, taking her hand in mine. She turned red eyes and a purple blotched nose towards the window and shook a fist in the direction of Miss Lilian's flat.

'It was that ginger tom of hers,' she sobbed. 'He must have slipped through the back door when I went to the dustbin, then hid himself somewhere until I let Billy out for his game of football.'

Billy was the name of the deceased. I had often watched him playing football. It was an astonishing sight. Released from the confines of the gleaming cage, he fluttered down on the table and took up his position on the touchline. Then wings aspan, he tore across to the other end of the table propelling a small celluloid ball along with his beak. He pulled up sharply in the penalty area and with great accuracy shot the ball between two tiny goal posts which Miss Coombe had set up before play commenced. After each goal scored he waited expectantly for his fans to clap; unless they did he hopped back into his cage and furiously attacked his cuttlefish, sulkily refusing to come out again. This made Miss Coombe very unhappy, and since it was a most important part of my duty to keep her happy I clapped heartily every time the little white ball went through the goal posts.

Now that poor Billy was no more I was glad that I had been unstinting with the applause. I would have cheered as well as clapped if he could have been restored to life.

I stayed with Miss Coombe until she was a little calmer, then I went to tell Miss Lilian about the awful thing Tommy had done to Billy. She was very upset, though not quite in the way I had expected. She viewed the tragedy from a different angle.

'What did she want to go letting it out of the cage for?' she asked crossly. 'Folks shouldn't keep birds if they can't look after them properly.' She gathered Tommy up in her arms. 'Diddums give him a nasty old budgie for his din-dins then?' she crooned, burying her face in his ginger fur. 'It would have served her right if you'd been sick on her carpet.' I left them together, feeling that in some inexplicable way I had got the boot entirely on the wrong foot, and should have been apologizing to Tommy instead of feeling sorry for Billy.

As Miss Lilian got older she became less and less capable of looking after herself. She sent home-helps away, saying that Tommy didn't like strange women in the house, and instead of spending her pension money, not to mention the windfall, on food and other things for her own wellbeing, she came back from the shops staggering under the weight of the goodies she had bought for her feline friend.

But Tommy had no appetite for the slices of raw liver, the uncooked steak and kidney, and the aromatic kippers which were spread for him on the floor. He got his fill from the birds and mice he caught while he was patrolling the grounds. Several times a day I went across to Miss Lilian's flat and picked up the tasty morsels which he had rejected but which the flies were attacking hungrily. As fast as I picked them up more were put down.

Meanwhile, the ginger cat was making himself increasingly unpopular with everybody round the Lodge. He gathered his harem on the rooftops at night and kept the residents awake with his orgiastic revellings; he threw the nice old gardener into a frenzy by going to the lavatory on the exact spot where the last lot of seeds had been sown, then threw him into another frenzy by fastidiously scraping the newly raked earth to hide his misdeeds; he also disappeared for days, making us wonder where he had gone, but unfortunately he always came back. It was about this time that I started asking the Lord whether, in some not too unkind way, He would rid me of the thorn that was beginning to pierce my flesh too sharply.

I had just begun to think that the plea had fallen on deaf ears when there came a knock at my door one Sunday morning. The man who had knocked stood nervously twiddling a crash helmet. His motorbike was propped up against the privet hedge.

'Sorry to trouble you,' he said. 'It was the matron I wanted.' After we had got over that little difficulty he told me what he wanted me for.

'It's the cat,' he said. 'The ginger tom that belongs to one of your old ladies.'

'What's happened to it?' I asked, trying not to sound too hopeful.

'He's dead,' he said. 'He shot straight under my front wheel. There wasn't a thing I could do about it. He's lying flat as a pancake out in the road.'

Because it was Sunday and neither the gardener nor the man who did the odd jobs was around to arrange the interment, I fetched a shovel from one of the sheds and the man scraped the flattened cat off the road. Then we walked solemnly down my path and out of the garden gate. I found a pleasant place under one of

Tommy's favourite trees and left the motor cyclist to do what he had to while I went to break the news to Miss Lilian.

She didn't hear me at first. She had grown very deaf and was busily arranging a few rather tired looking slices of boiled ham on the carpet. There was a saucerful of milk and two sardines on a plate to add variety to Tommy's lunch.

'I'm afraid I've got some bad news for you,' I shouted. 'Tommy's just been run over.' I expected her to collapse at my feet in a huddle of inconsolable grief but she did nothing of the sort. She rearranged the ham, shifted the saucer of milk a little to the left and stepped back to make sure that all was as Tommy would expect it to be when he came in for lunch.

'Ah well, what is to be will be, I suppose,' she said, and added another sardine from the tin on the dresser. Relieved as I was that there had been no hysterics I was a little surprised at her calm acceptance of the blow I had dealt her.

'Would you like to come to the garden and watch him being buried?' I asked in a high pitched shriek. After I had said it twice she nodded and took off her pinny, then thought better of it and put it back on again. She put on her hat and coat, changed her shoes, took a clean handkerchief out of the dresser drawer and a handbag from the little cupboard by the side of the fireplace, and we walked to where the motorcyclist was standing in an attitude of respect for the dead. He muttered a few words of condolence into one of her deaf ears and proceeded with the burial.

Tommy strolled up just as we were scattering rose petals on his grave. He rubbed himself against the man's water-proofed legs, purring loudly, sniffed at the newly dug mound of earth and went off home with Miss Lilian, who had already forgotten what she had gone there for in the first place, if she had ever known.

I never discovered who owned the ginger cat that had been buried with due reverence under one of Tommy's favourite trees, but oddly enough I was glad it wasn't him. However fervently I may have prayed for his dispatch, there was something rather worrying about prayers being answered in such a drastic way. He was to be a thorn in my flesh for a little longer.

After the third occasion that a policeman had found Miss Lilian wandering around the town in the middle of the night with her faithful friend trailing behind on the end of a long piece of rope, it was reluctantly decided that she would have to go somewhere more suited to her needs. I packed her few belongings, tried over and over again to tell her what was happening and went with her to the hospital where she was to stay for the rest of her life. Then I went back to the Lodge to think what should be done about Tommy.

For a time I thought the problem was solved. When he realized that there was no response to his pitiful cries at the door of the flat that had once been his home, he disappeared and wasn't seen for several days. The day he came back was a memorable one.

Miss Coombe still hadn't quite recovered from the loss of her budgerigar when she returned from an overnight stay with a friend, found her flat in a state of chaos and Tommy crouched on the table ready to spring. He also had had an overnight stay.

Miss Coombe screamed, neighbours rushed from every side to see what was happening and Tommy streaked along the verandah and was at my gate just as I opened it to find out why all the emergency bells were ringing at once. He was sitting in my apple tree when I got back from doing what I could for poor Miss Coombe.

Seeing him sitting there, washing his whiskers as if nothing had happened, filled me with such fury that I decided to answer my prayers for his dispatch myself. I flew at the tree, he flew down it and took refuge in my dustbin, the lid of which had been left off. I imprisoned him in the bin and waited for somebody to come to my aid.

It was the gardener who heard my cries for help. He took over with the dustbin lid while I telephoned the RSPCA. Two men arrived wearing strong leather gloves and went off with Tommy in their van.

I never saw him again. I told the committee what had happened and begged them in future never to weaken when an applicant for one of the flatlets turned up at the interview with a heaving cat basket.

Chapter Nine

BECAUSE THE AVERAGE age of the residents was round about seventy it wasn't to be expected that romance would play a significant part in their lives. The pangs of unrequited love had been buried deep with other painful little pangs, and a cuddle in the dark was something to be frowned on when young couples, who were supposed to be watching the film, sat with their heads so close together that they obstructed the view of the more single-minded picturegoers.

Those who had once been married might occasionally look back with a sigh, remembering the days when a peck on the cheek was enough to send a tingle down the spine, and nights when there had been another pair of feet in bed to make a hot water bottle unnecessary. But usually they had become reconciled to the hot water bottle before they came to live at the Lodge, or made a brave attempt at looking as if they had.

The residents who had never been married, and shouldn't by rights have had any memories about more than one pair of feet in their beds, surprised me sometimes with stories of young love that would have sent their mothers to an early grave if they'd had any inkling of what was going on. But those who had stayed single for whatever reason seemed to have lost any regrets they might once have had at missing out on the ups and downs of marriage.

Except for Miss Bains who had shocked her critics by getting married when they thought she should have been preparing herself for Higher Things, nobody had set tongues wagging on the verandah until Gladys Smythe started courting. As was to be expected, it was Mrs Turgoose who gave me the details of the romance.

Mrs Turgoose had been keeping me informed of the scandals that were currently rocking the senior citizens' clubs since the day I went to work at the Lodge. I got many a dig in the ribs while she was telling me of the underhand things that went on at the domino drives, and the low tricks the whist players resorted to in order to win the quarter of tea or the pot of home-made jam for holding the highest scoring card.

Her accounts were particularly venomous after she or her partner had been caught red-handed in the act of revoking, or had been beaten by foul means rather than fair, as was often the case according to Mrs Turgoose.

'They'd never have won if he hadn't kept winking at her to tell her to lead low,' she snarled after she and her partner had suffered a particularly humiliating defeat when a quarter of tea and a pot of home-made rhubarb and ginger jam had been fought over with grim determination. 'And if he'd had a spark of decency in him he'd have refused the prize he got for winning the raffle. He should have been satisfied with the pot of jam without taking the bottle of lavender water as well.' Apparently Mrs Turgoose had set her heart on winning the lavender water which the warden of the club had graciously presented to the man whose raffle ticket was the first to be drawn, having already presented him with the pot of jam for being smarter at whist than Mrs Turgoose. 'And what any man wants with a bottle of scent I hardly like to think.'

'Perhaps he wanted it to give to the lady he kept winking at,' I said. Mrs Turgoose treated the flippancy with the contempt it merited.

'I wouldn't care if it stopped at winking during whist drives,' she went on, 'but I saw him with my own two eyes put his hands on his partner's knee one afternoon when they were playing draughts.' I allowed my eyebrows to rise almost as far as my hair line. 'Mind you,' continued Mrs Turgoose, 'I have to say in fairness to them both that they're man and wife, but there's a time and place for everything and a game of draughts needs all your concentration if you're not going to be huffed all the time.' Though I didn't know what being huffed meant I could see by Mrs Turgoose's face that it was something to be avoided.

On the Monday morning that Mrs Turgoose told me the news about Mrs Smythe's romance she opened her door to me bubbling with excitement.

'Come in quick,' she said, 'I've got something to tell you.' I picked my way through the perennials that were waiting to be thrown in the washtub and sat down, almost as excited as she was. Whatever squeamishness I might once have had about listening to gossip had been finally quashed after I had persuaded myself that there was no harm in listening to it so long as I didn't rush out at breakneck speed to pass it on to others. This was something which the sister tutor at my training school had tried to warn us against. 'Never pass on to a friend a secret that has just been passed on to you,' she had said in the middle of a lecture one day. 'It is well to remember that thy friend hath a friend.' As well as being a Quaker, our sister tutor was a very wise lady. We might have benefited more from her teachings if we had listened harder. But remembering her words had often stopped me when I was on the point of opening my mouth when I should have kept it closed. Indiscretions have a way of going round in full circle.

Mrs Turgoose kept me waiting in suspense while she threw the flowers into the suds, then she brought two cups of tea into the living room and sat down.

'Gladys Smythe's courting,' she said.

'Which Gladys Smythe?' I asked, as if the Lodge was crawling with ladies of that unlikely name.

'Her upstairs. The one that's my best friend,' said Mrs Turgoose with justifiable impatience. I stared at her.

'I don't believe it,' I said. I didn't believe it. Mrs Smythe was the last person in the world I would have expected to hear was courting. She was plump like Mrs Turgoose, though an inch or two taller, with the same snowy white hair befitting her three score years and ten, and a few more besides if the dates on her tattered old baptismal certificate were to be believed. She had come to live at the Lodge after her husband died suddenly when they were sitting on the pier at Blackpool. They had gone on an old folk's outing. Mrs Turgoose was with them when it happened. She said that it had quite spoilt the illuminations for her. But it hadn't spoilt her long friendship with Mrs Smythe; if anything it had strengthened it. She had put in a good word with the committee when she applied for one of the flats and had given her a hand with filling in the forms. For, as Mrs Turgoose said, 'a friend in need is a friend indeed', and with no wish to blow her own trumpet she was never backward in coming forward when it came to doing a good turn for a friend.

'Who's she courting?' I asked, after Mrs Turgoose had assured me that whether I believed it or not was neither here nor there. It was a fact, may she never move again.

'It's somebody she got pally with while she was helping on menswear at the Labour Party Jumble Sale,' said Mrs Turgoose, looking suitably gratified that her latest bit of gossip had found such an appreciative audience. She knew I had been a nurse for a long time and it took a lot to startle me. I was well and truly startled.

Mrs Smythe and Mrs Turgoose were loyal supporters of the local Labour Party. They regularly attended meetings at the Cooperative Hall and spoke in disparaging terms of the Tories and Liberals who infiltrated the citizens' senior club, to which they both belonged. They wore their rosettes with pride while they were handing out leaflets when an election was imminent, and sang the paean of praise to the Red

Flag in thanksgiving when their member was returned. If their member wasn't returned they blamed the electorate for being gullible and predicted all sorts of terrible troubles with the Tories in power. It was a foregone conclusion that nobody but a staunch Labour supporter would have stood a chance with Mrs Smythe. Sir Winston might have tilted the scales slightly, but he had gone the way of her husband, though not, of course, while sitting on the pier at Blackpool.

Mrs Turgoose told me that the man at the Labour Party Jumble Sale had had his eye on Gladys Smythe for a long time – or so he said. But nothing had come of it until he went to buy a couple of nearly new shirts at the stall she was on. After he'd bought the shirts he'd decided to buy a pair of trousers, and not being sure of his waist measurements, he'd asked Mrs Smythe if she would mind running a tape measure round him. She'd still got both arms round his ample waist when he happened to mention that she reminded him in a lot of ways of his good wife who had passed away shortly after the war. Mrs Smythe had got so flustered when he told her this that she'd had to put the tape round again to make sure she'd got the measurements right. And that was that, said Mrs Turgoose. The next thing they knew he'd joined the Darby and Joan club, and soon he and Mrs Smythe were playing dominoes every afternoon, or sitting side by side doing a crossword puzzle. Mrs Turgoose said she'd always done the crossword puzzle with her friend but she'd had her nose pushed out of joint. Not that she minded, she said, sounding as if she minded very much, she'd never been one to intrude where she wasn't wanted.

To anybody who wasn't aware of the flame that had been kindled in Mrs Smythe's motherly bosom she looked no different, on the surface, from the way she had always looked. There was nothing to suggest that she had suddenly been transported to the Seventh Inn of Happiness. It was only because I had been told her secret that I thought I detected a faint flush on her cheeks and a slight hesitation in her voice when she told me, while I was doing the round one day, that she had invited a friend for tea if I had no objections. From the way she avoided my eye I was left in no doubt that the friend who was coming to tea was the man who had kindled the flame. I was only too happy that he was coming for tea. Nevertheless I decided not to make things too easy for her.

'Of course I haven't any objections,' I said heartily. 'Which friend have you invited? Do I know her?' Mrs Smythe smoothed her pinny, patted her already immaculate hair, and showed every sign of being an extremely embarrassed lady.

'Well, no,' she said, flicking an imaginary speck of dust off the table. 'I don't think you've met her, I mean him.' She stopped, then started again. 'As a matter of fact it's a man, not a woman.' Having got over that little hurdle she relaxed slightly and waited for me to take things a step further.

'Oh, now isn't that nice,' I burbled. 'A friend of the family is he?' The little flush came back to Mrs Smythe's cheeks and she stooped to fiddle with her shoelace.

'Well, not exactly,' she said, then went on to tell me about the events that had led to her inviting a gentleman friend for tea. It took her as long as it had taken Mrs Turgoose, but not by so much as a look did I reveal that I had heard it all before. I was quite dewy eyed when I eventually left her. She had already got her mixing bowl out and was preparing to make a cake, a few jam tarts and a batch of scones. If the way to a man's heart was via his digestive system she was determined that the distance should be as short as possible.

That afternoon I made it my business to be strolling along the verandah when the gentleman friend arrived. He was a well-built man and I understood exactly why Mrs Smythe had to put both arms round his waist when she was measuring him for the trousers. She would have had to stand on tip-toes as well.

He was carrying a large bunch of flowers which looked as if they had been freshly picked from his garden or allotment. From the way he held them it wasn't difficult to guess that it had been a long time since he had taken flowers to a lady. Their heads were trailing almost to the ground and they seemed to be tied up with enough string to stretch from one end of a row of beans to the other.

As I stood in the shadows of the porch watching his progress across the forecourt I earnestly hoped that he wouldn't raise his eyes to any of the windows. It wasn't every day that a gentleman came calling on one of the residents. I knew I wouldn't be the only one who was watching the scene with interest.

For a time the courtship was confined to a weekly visit, a cup of tea, and a selection of home-baked goodies to prove that Mrs Smythe could cook. Then came the day when the lady was seen walking arm in arm with her friend on the way to the Darby and Joan club. It was a touching sight, or so I thought, choking back a sob. But not everybody shared my sentiments.

'Well, all I can say is that there's no fool like an old fool,' said Mrs Marsh, who was standing beside me at

Mrs Beauchamp's window watching the happy pair. 'They'll be getting spliced next, I shouldn't wonder.'

'But they're spliced already, and have been for a long time,' said Mrs Beauchamp, who had picked up a lot of slang words from her friend and whose mind wandered to her erring husband and Florence whenever anything implying marriage was mentioned. 'Don't you remember, dear? I've told you so often how Mr Beauchamp had to go to that dreadful hotel in Brighton with a young woman he'd never seen before in his life so that we could be divorced without poor Florence's name being dragged in the mud. The young woman was sent from some sort of agency and he allowed her to sleep in the bed while he sat in a chair. So considerate of him I always thought.'

'Oh Gawd, she's off again,' said Mrs Marsh turning from the window and touching her head meaningfully. 'It's Gladys Smythe and her bloke I'm talking about, not your ex and his bird. And if you believe that old rubbish about him sitting in a chair all night you'd believe anything. There isn't a man in the world that would sit in a chair all night if there was a bed handy and a woman willing to get in it with him. It wouldn't be natural. Men are men, whether they're toffs like your old man or a bit of a rough diamond like my Harry was. Unless, of course, we're talking about monks, or them chaps you read about that's supposed to put powder and stuff on their faces. But your old man couldn't have been one of them 'cos if he had been you wouldn't have had your Evelyn.'

'Yes, dear,' said Mrs Beauchamp, who hadn't understood a word.

I was greatly indebted to Mrs Turgoose for her progress report on her friend's courtship. I was indebted to her for all the snippets of information which kept me in touch with current affairs. Without them I would have remained in ignorance of much that was going on around me.

'They've started going for nine pennyworth of dark in the pictures on Monday afternoons,' she told me when we were peeping at the couple through the see-through net curtains that had recently replaced the heavier Nottingham lace.

When she saw that I wasn't too sure what was meant by nine pennyworth of dark in the pictures she hastened to explain.

'Pensioners get in for ninepence in the afternoon. It costs double to go at night. Glad says he pays for them to get in but she pays for the ice cream in the interval. She's like me, Glad is. Generous to a fault.'

The courtship went from strength to strength. There were visits to stately homes and gardens, coach trips to the seaside – but never of course to Blackpool – that would have stirred up too many memories for Mrs Smythe; and finally there was a week at a holiday camp laid on by one of the local organizations in the off-peak period. Mrs Turgoose told me that her friend hadn't been able to make up her mind about that for a long time. She was worried there might be gossip, seeing that her gentleman friend was going as well. But Mrs Turgoose had reminded her that there had been plenty of gossip already so a bit more wouldn't hurt her. In the end Mrs Smythe appended her name to the list and paid the deposit.

In spite of the organizers of the holiday insisting on the sexes being segregated prompt at ten every night, just as at my training school, there was plenty of opportunity for the courting couple to get better acquainted. They had strolls along the esplanade and pier, their usual nine pennyworth of dark in the pictures on the Monday afternoon, and got free tickets for the Winter Garden show. When it was all over Mrs Smythe came home with a faraway look in her eyes.

'What's wrong with her?' I asked Mrs Turgoose when the look persisted into another week. 'She hasn't been the same woman since she came back from the holiday camp. Did it rain every day, or was the food terrible?' I knew that either could ruin a holiday. I had occasionally had holidays ruined by a combination of both.

'No, it's nothing like that,' replied Mrs Turgoose. 'As far as I know a good time was had by all, except for one or two of them going down with the collywobbles through eating winkles that wasn't fresh as they might have been.' I had never touched a winkle. They had been on my mother's list of forbidden foods. Whenever we went to Skegness on choir outings she had made me have bread and jam for tea, instead of the selection of shellfish which the more adventurous choristers were sampling at the expense of the church. My mother was the same about Gorgonzola cheese. She had turned me against it at an early age. Her description of the maggots which she said it was alive with was enough to turn anybody against it.

'Then what *is* the matter with Mrs Smythe?' I asked. Mrs Turgoose glanced round the flat as if afraid that the walls might have had ears, then she leaned forward and spoke in a hoarse whisper. I had to lean forward to catch what she was saying.

'She wants to get married,' she said. I leaned back, relieved that there was nothing more for me to worry about.

I wasn't surprised that Mrs Smythe wanted to get married. With all the little outings she'd been enjoying, not to mention the week at the holiday camp, she must have reached the stage when she wanted some official recognition.

'Then why don't they get married?' I asked, as if there was no more to getting married than naming the day. Mrs Turgoose leaned forward again.

'It's his son. The one he lives with. He's a bachelor and a bit set in his ways, him being not far off sixty. He's always been strict with his dad and won't hear of him getting married again. He won't even let him take Glad home for a cup of tea when they've been to the pictures. That's why she always has to bring him back here.' I could hardly believe my ears. This was a different slant on the so-called generation gap we were starting to hear so much about.

'And it's not only that,' Mrs Turgoose continued. 'Even if they did get married, they wouldn't be as well off as they are now. Two separate pensions is more than a married couple gets. The only way they'd be as well off would be for them to live in sin and Glad would never stand for that. She's always kept herself respectable has Glad.' I had no doubt that Glad had. She would hardly want to spoil the record at her time of life.

The faraway look in Mrs Smythe's eyes gradually went, but when it was finally accepted by both parties that her gentleman friend's son was never going to give his consent to the marriage there were no dramatic farewell scenes, and no bitter casting up of promises made under the light of an early moon at the holiday camp. Instead, the courtship settled down into a placid, comfortable friendship which neither the charitable body nor the Social Security watchdogs could have taken exception to. On Mondays Mr Jones came to call for Mrs Smythe to go to the pictures. When the big film was over and they had sat through the adverts and newsreel again she brought him back to her flat and gave him a large enough meal to make him loosen his belt at the end of it. On high days and holidays they took a flask of tea and a bite of something to eat and went for a bus ride; they even went for a day at the seaside in the summer, but they never went back to the holiday camp.

It was Mrs Turgoose who told me that her friend's friend's name was Mr Jones. Mrs Smythe never referred to him as anything but 'my friend', and she even said that rather shyly.

After Mr Jones had stopped being a bashful suitor, and become just a good friend instead, he brought other things as well as flowers when he came to visit Mrs Smythe. He arrived with bags full of potatoes, arms full of cabbages and hands full of runner beans, and other things his allotment brought forth in their due season. The produce was distributed amongst the residents in order of Mrs Smythe's preference.

'She's already had one cabbage this week,' said Mrs Turgoose huffily when she saw another being delivered to Miss Coombe's door. 'I never seem to get a look in with the cabbages.' She told me that apparently Mr Jones's son didn't approve of his father being so generous with the vegetables, but for once Mr Jones had asserted himself. He told his son that since it was he who grew the stuff he had a perfect right to dispose of it in whatever way he wished. Mrs Turgoose said that he hadn't put it quite like that but that was what he had meant. I thought it was a pity that Mr Jones hadn't asserted himself sooner, especially in the matter of getting married again, but as it turned out it was just as well he hadn't. Mrs Smythe would have been a widow again before the next spring greens were ready for cutting.

The first intimation I got that all was not as it should be with Mr Jones was when Mrs Smythe rang her bell soon after lunch one Monday afternoon. I spent a few moments wondering if it was a false alarm. She hadn't looked as if she was sickening for anything when I visited her that morning, and had gone into some detail about the film she and her friend were going to see, saying that it was one that she had been wanting to see for a long time. It was a warm, sunny day, and just right for a gentle stroll through the park and to the pictures. Then I stopped wondering and went across as quickly as I could without breaking into a run and causing panic amongst the residents.

As was usual after a bell had been rung anxious little groups stood on the verandah speculating on whether whoever had rung it would need a doctor, an ambulance, or at the worst a hearse. I pushed my way past them and hurried up the stairs. Mrs Smythe was waiting for me at the door. Her face was ashen.

'It's him,' she gasped. 'I think he's gone.' Ignoring the rule that forbids nurses to run except in the case of fire or haemorrhage, I ran into the room. Mr Jones was sitting in an armchair with his head resting on the antimacassar. His eyes were closed and he was as ashen as Mrs Smythe. I felt for his pulse: it was beating fairly steadily.

'I told you he'd gone,' wailed Mrs Smythe, pacing the room and wringing her hands. Mr Jones opened his eyes and glared at her.

'Of course I ain't gone, you silly old cow,' he said, lifting his head from the antimacassar. I was delighted to hear that they were still close enough for him to feel free to address her in such endearing terms. I was also delighted that he had the strength to make such a vehement statement. Mrs Smythe stopped pacing the room. She was almost back to her normal colour.

'Then why were you lolling back in the chair with your eyes shut?' she demanded, standing over him and returning glare for glare. 'It was enough to frighten anybody to death seeing you looking like that.' Mr Jones shook his head vigorously, blinked hard a few times then rolled up his trouser legs. Mrs Smythe looked away modestly.

'I was having one of me turns,' he said, briskly rubbing the exposed legs to restore the circulation.

'It's the first I've heard about you having turns,' said Mrs Smythe, still with her eyes averted.

'It wouldn't do to tell you everything,' he said, rolling down his trouser legs, and giving her a nice little smile. 'You'd only start to worry, and think you'd got to mollycoddle me. If there's anything I can't abide it's being mollycoddled.' Mrs Smythe went off to put the kettle on. When she came back she patted her friend's hand to let him know that all was forgiven.

After we had all had a cup of tea I suggested that instead of going to the pictures they should play Scrabble. Which they did.

The next time Mr Jones had one of his turns he didn't have to be mollycoddled. The day that his son took him his early morning cup of tea and found the late night cup of cocoa still on his bed table and very cold, he informed friends and relations that his father was dead. Unfortunately he didn't inform Mrs Smythe. She only found out the next day after Mrs Turgoose heard about it when she was doing her shopping.

Mrs Smythe wasn't invited to the funeral either, and though she sent a wreath, 'From Glad with Love', it wasn't mentioned in the acknowledgements in the local paper. Nobody would have guessed she had been the old man's closest friend for the past three years.

'I think it's diabolical the way she's been treated,' said Mrs Turgoose. I had to agree.

Mrs Smythe aged very much over the next few months. She often made do with a tin of soup for lunch instead of cooking the savoury little meals that had made my mouth water if I was late doing the round. She left the bit of smoked haddock she had bought for her tea untouched, and didn't have a baking day any more. She stopped having her hair set once a week and didn't even bother to put on a clean pinny every afternoon.

'That woman's going all to pieces,' said Mrs Turgoose. 'She won't be here much longer if she doesn't pull herself together.'

But it wasn't the loss of appetite, or the fact that she

didn't have her hair set regularly that told me how much Mrs Smythe missed her gentleman friend. It was something far more poignant.

I went into her flat one morning and looked round wondering what had happened to it. There were still four chairs and a table as there had always been, there was the rag rug that she had pegged herself, and the little bed that took up the wall behind the dividing curtains. There was the dresser with cups hanging from hooks, and plates and saucers arranged on the shelves, but there was something missing, and at first I didn't know what it was.

'What have you done to your room?' I asked, looking round in bewilderment. 'There seems to be something missing.'

'There is,' she said wearily. 'I've got rid of all his things.'

'What things?' I asked, still not understanding.

'All the things he's given me over the years. I couldn't stand seeing them any more so I've pushed them away in the cupboard.' And then I knew. Gone was the little striped tiger and the tiny koala bear which had stood side by side on her dresser since a trip to the zoo in the early days of the courtship. Gone the china cats and dogs, the miniature milk jugs and teapots with 'A Present from Margate' scrawled in gold lettering. Saddest of all, gone was the framed snapshot of Mrs Smythe and Mr Jones that somebody had taken while they were posing on the pier at Clacton. There wasn't a thing left to remind her of the happy days they had spent together.

'But you shouldn't have done it,' I said, sitting beside her and trying not to look at the empty spaces. 'You'll have nothing to remember him by.'

'That's why I did it,' she said. 'Maybe now I can't see them I shall stop remembering the days he bought them. I might even stop thinking about him as much as I've been doing.'

But she didn't stop thinking about him. Mrs Turgoose gave her a few plastic flowers to fill the gaps on the dresser but it was a long time before she could be persuaded to help on the menswear stall at the Labour Party Jumble Sale. As Mrs Turgoose said, 'She could have ended up dying of a broken heart if it hadn't been for me taking her out of herself and making her volunteer for menswear at the meeting.' I didn't argue with her. I knew because I was a nurse that nobody dies of a broken heart, but because I was a woman I knew that the heart can play some very funny tricks.

Part Three

Part Three

Chapter Ten

THERE ARE MANY words in the English language that are used to describe the frailties of man – and of woman as well, of course. Some are less kind than others and some spring to mind more often when adjectives are needed to paint a picture of an aged one who has grown old less than gracefully. Mrs Peters, who moved in shortly after Miss Lilian and her cat had gone, hadn't grown old gracefully at all. From the things I heard before she moved in she had never been noted for her endearing qualities, and over the years she had got more stubborn, crotchety and difficult than she had even been in her younger days. By the time she was drawing her old age pension she had earned quite a number of the uncomplimentary things that were said about her behind her back.

After her husband died, henpecked to the end it was rumoured, she had sold the house, gloated over the price she had extorted from the buyer and, thereafter, until she came to live at the Lodge, had devoted herself to her family on a rotation system, one branch having the pleasure of her company for three long months before she moved on to plague the life out of another. It often took the rest of the year while she wasn't in residence to repair the damage she did during the months of togetherness. She was able to set sister against brother, husband against wife, and half the next generation at each other's throats simply by appearing on the doorstep with her luggage.

But in spite of the knack she had of arousing their worst feelings, none of her children seemed overjoyed at the thought of her coming to live at the Lodge.

'It isn't that we don't want her,' protested a son, with guilt emblazoned on his face. 'Or that we don't love her,' chimed in a daughter, showing by her anxiety how much she loved her mother. 'It's just that what-ever we do is wrong when she's staying with us. If she isn't carping at the children she's grumbling at us, and telling me how the housekeeping money should be spent. And she practically takes over in the kitchen the moment she sets foot in the house.'

They didn't need to protest to me. I had known for a long time that however good the intentions were it wasn't easy for two or three generations to live in close harmony for more than a very limited period. I had heard stories while I was a nurse in hospital that had made me less inclined to condemn families who for one reason or another were reluctant to take in an aged parent as a permanent guest. A patient I once nursed had told me that her mother had moved in with her and her husband shortly after they got married and was still occupying the spare room on her ninetieth birthday. The patient had sounded very bitter when she was telling me that ever so many people at the party had said that her mother looked as young as she did. Allowing for a bit of exaggeration I could see why. A long-term triangular arrangement like that must have put a great strain on the husband and wife. Having Mrs Peters in the spare room even for three months must have put a strain on her family. It wasn't easy for me having her as a permanent resident.

I had my first brush with the new resident on the day she moved in; it was the forerunner of many.

'Hello, dear,' I said brightly, when I went across to find out if there was anything she needed. 'I hope everything is to your satisfaction.' Nothing was to her satisfaction, either then or at any other time. She glared at me and I shrank back. I had never been a brave woman and I wasn't a brave matron. Anybody as forceful as Mrs Peters could reduce me to shreds.

'The cooker doesn't work, the tap's got a drip and

there's a nasty smell coming from somewhere,' she said without drawing breath. I knew at once that her family had done well to warn me that mother could be difficult at times.

It took me longer than a few minutes to investigate Mrs Peters' complaints, and to promise her that they would be dealt with at the odd job man's earliest convenience, and when she insisted that his earliest convenience should be there and then, I rushed off to look for him. With her standing over him directing operations he worked faster than I had ever seen him work before. When at last the tap wasn't dripping, the fault in the cooker had been corrected (she hadn't turned it on at the mains) and every manhole in the grounds had been lifted to prove that the nasty smell wasn't coming from there, I made a mental note to censor the report I put in to the committee. Mrs Peters had said some very cutting things while the work was being done, none of which would have looked well in print.

I was about to leave the room after rather belatedly wishing her every happiness in her new home when I noticed a carving knife and fork lying on the lino just beneath her bed. I stooped and picked them up, mistakenly thinking that this was just the opportunity I needed to restore Mrs Peters' confidence in me. It had been quite badly shaken while I was investigating her complaints.

'Why, look what I've found under the bed,' I cried gaily. 'They must have dropped out of one of the packing cases.' Before I had time to take the cutlery across to the dresser where I thought it belonged Mrs Peters snatched it off me.

'You leave them alone,' she said angrily. 'They're there for a purpose and I'll thank you not to interfere with them. I doubt whether they'll work now with you messing about with them.' She dropped on her knees and placed the knife and fork exactly as they were before I disturbed them.

'What are they there for?' I ventured to ask.

'They're for warding off the cramp,' she said, getting up from her knees. 'I used to get it every night until somebody told me that keeping a knife and fork under the bed drives it away. But they have to be put down properly or else they don't work.'

Though I had never had any faith in such charms myself, I knew a lot of people who did. My mother had firmly believed that a lump of steak buried in the garden would banish the most persistent warts. But as none of us had ever had warts she never got the chance to prove it.

It wasn't until much later when I was making Mrs

Peters' bed one morning (she was feeling too liverish to make it herself) that I found evidence to suggest that she didn't rely entirely on the magical power of the cutlery. Tucked between the sheets at the bottom of the bed, with a corn pad or two and a few wisps of chiropodist's floss, were three small and wizened nutmegs. I replaced them carefully after I had turned the mattress, terrified that they might lose some of their potency through being handled by an unbeliever.

Neither did I lay too many infidel fingers on the dried-up potato which she kept under her pillow as a talisman. From the smell of embrocation which I occasionally detected in the flat I suspected that the talisman didn't always work. But I never voiced my suspicions.

Miss Lilian's flat had been empty for quite a few weeks when Mrs Peters began stepping up her complaints about the one she was in. But as well as finding fresh faults with the cooker, and insisting that there was a dead rat under the floorboards causing the nasty smell, she began to falter a little when she was walking along the verandah to her door, even stumbling slightly so long as she could be sure there was somebody near enough to see that she didn't actually fall. Those who watched from their windows reported that they had seen her holding onto the wall and gasping for breath, and those who were willing to listen were told that the long walk along the verandah to her door would be the death of her one of these days.

It was no coincidence that the flatlet which Miss Lilian and her cat had left empty was in the process of being redecorated throughout, and would soon be ready for a new tenant; sweet, clean and wholesome, with bright new wallpaper, fresh paint, and not a hint of Tommy left. Mrs Peters had quite made up her mind to be its new tenant, exchanging the somewhat jaded decor of Flat 16 for the splendours of Flat 4a.

There were, however, certain formalities before such an exchange could be made. The formalities included supplying the committee with enough evidence that the transfer was necessary. It was with this in mind that Mrs Peters allowed her feet to falter almost to stumbling point, and her breath to come in short pants whenever she had an audience while she was walking along the verandah.

From the rumours I heard when I was doing the rounds she had lost none of her agility, or strength to draw breath, when she thought she wasn't being watched. She walked briskly up the street with her shopping basket and pushed to the front of the queues for anything that was in short supply or on special offer. She rampaged round the supermarket tearing off price labels that had only been stuck on that morning, refusing to pay a penny more than the price of the day before. She examined eggs for hairline cracks, and stuck her fingers deep into fruit to test for ripeness. She tapped her foot impatiently while the girl who was serving her in the shoe shop climbed up and down ladders with an assortment of colours, shapes and sizes, then, head high and face black with anger, she stormed out saying that she would go somewhere else for her shoes, where the service was better and there was a wider choice. Nobody who had once served Mrs Peters fell over themselves to serve her again.

But it was a surprisingly meek lady who approached me one morning with the proposition that she should be allowed to move into the empty flat. I hardly recognized the sweet-faced old thing who invited me in and begged me to have a cup of tea. I had never had a cup of tea with Mrs Peters.

She didn't come to the point at once. Uncharacteristically she asked me how my family was, wiped away a tear at the mention of my new little granddaughter, gave me another cup of tea, then popped the question.

'But why do you want to move?' I asked her. 'You haven't lived here long and this flat is no different from the empty one.' I could almost hear her thinking that being newly decorated made the empty one very different. She clutched at the front of her blouse.

'It's the breathing you see,' she wheezed, struggling hard to follow one breath with the next. 'And the legs aren't as good as they were.' She took a few tottering steps across the room, gripping the table for support. 'This flat's too far along the verandah for me to walk to every time I go out. I need the one on the other side that's nearer the door.' She flopped back in her chair, indicating that the few tottering steps would be as much as she could manage that day.

'But there's a door on this side you could use,' I said. 'You don't have to walk all the way round.' She breathed heavily for a moment or two while she thought what line to take next.

'It's the heart,' she said, pursing her lips in an effort to turn them blue. 'And the nerves.' She let her hand shake in a very nervous way. 'I've never been right since the moment I stepped inside this flat. There's something about it that doesn't agree with me. I shan't be here much longer unless they let me move.' I looked round the flat. It was very pleasant. It contained, among other things, a neat little chintz-covered sofa, a rocking chair, and a very old gate-legged table. There was also a Victorian love seat and a collection of figurines and small objects that had been handed down or given as presents a long time ago.

The love seat was beautiful. I had never seen one before. The two chairs were united in the middle, each facing in opposite directions. Despite its name it would have been well nigh impossible for whoever was sitting in the chairs to have even held hands. Any other demonstration of affection would have been as difficult to achieve as the most straight-laced Victorian parent could have wished. Which no doubt was what the craftsman had in mind when he fashioned the love seat.

Three of the little porcelain figures that were arranged on the mantelpiece were to disappear before Mrs Peters moved into Flat 4a. When I read in an article on antiques that they were German fairings and much sought after by collectors I raced across to tell Mrs Peters she was rich. I was too late. There were three little spaces where the German fairings had been.

'Where are they?' I asked her.

'I sold them yesterday,' she said. 'Two nice young men knocked at the door and asked if I had any old junk to sell. They wanted the love seat, but I said it was spoken for after I'd gone, so they said that seeing as I was an old lady and not very well off, they'd give me a fiver for the "Last in bed put out the light" things. I never liked them much anyway. The old woman in bed, and the old man with his night shirt on blowing out the candle, didn't seem the right sort of ornament to have on the mantelpiece. Anyway they were only given away at fairs for knocking coconuts off so I knew they couldn't be worth much. I took the fiver quick before the two young men changed their mind. It'll come in handy when I go to the seaside on one of the outings.'

I swallowed hard and went back home. There seemed no point in telling her that the little porcelain people preparing for bed were worth a great deal more than a day at the seaside. I was glad she hadn't let the nice young men buy the love seat, even if they had offered her enough to pay for a whole week at the seaside.

I never let anybody be robbed like that again. I warned all the residents that in future if two nice young men called and offered to buy their bric-a-brac they were to shut their doors and ring for me. If the young men turned out to be genuine I would still be there to see fair play.

It was Mrs Peters' doctor who finally got her into Flat 4a. He had been her doctor long enough to know that once she had set her heart on getting something she wore everybody down until she got it. After one or two half-hearted attempts at telling her that she wasn't in danger of dying if she didn't get the transfer, he wrote out a certificate with enough undecipherable words to impress the committee, and in due course the letter arrived giving her permission to move.

The effect on her health was miraculous. No sooner had she read the letter than she took a deep breath, shook off all the former ills that had rendered her almost helpless, and walked briskly along the verandah to inspect her future home.

I congratulated her on the good news and marvelled that anybody could wield such power. When I rang the family to ask them how she did it they said that it came from years of practice. Her methods had never been known to fail. First she ranted, then she raved, then if neither the ranting nor raving had the desired effect, she clutched the front of her blouse and tottered around, saying in faltering tones that they'd all be sorry when she was in her grave, sent there no doubt by their ingratitude. Since nobody was willing to take the responsibility for killing her she had managed to get her own way and stay alive.

She was a great help on the day she moved. The legs that had so often threatened to buckle beneath her strode purposefully backwards and forwards, while she carried pots and pans, objets d'art and bric-a-brac from the flat she was leaving to the flat she had schemed so hard to move to. The breathing that had been such a burden to her was now easy enough to let her make the many journeys with no stress at all. She stood first in one flat and then the other while the old gardener, the young odd job man, and middle-aged me, staggered with the three-piece suite, the rocking chair and all the other removables. On her instructions we put things here, there and everywhere, and every time she changed her mind we moved them all around until they were in entirely different places. The reason it had been left to us to do the moving was because somebody's grandmother had died and all Mrs Peters' relations were going to the funeral. The old gardener said he didn't believe a word of it and even I was a bit suspicious. But we both agreed that in their shoes we'd probably have done the same.

After the little love seat had been moved to a dozen different places, and when the last bit of bric-a-brac was where she wanted it to be, Mrs Peters looked round the flat with a critical eye. 'The wallpaper doesn't exactly match the carpet, does it?' she said. My heart sank. For somebody as pernickety as Mrs Peters, having wallpaper that didn't match the carpet could be the start of another war. I told her that in my opinion the pink in the carpet picked out the green in the wallpaper very nicely. But even as I was saying it I had the feeling that I was wasting my breath.

When the charitable body decided at one of their meetings that the time had come to make a few changes round the Lodge, the scheme was started in a modest way. The old-fashioned ranges with the mirrored overmantels were to be torn out and replaced with nice little characterless tiled fireplaces; cupboards and shelves, and all other fixtures and fittings that had given faithful service for nearly seventy years were to be renewed, and various other small things done to make the Lodge less of a Victorian relic. But all this took money and the charitable body hadn't an unlimited supply. It was therefore agreed that the work should be done in easy stages, starting with the flat which Mrs Peters had just vacated. After that it would continue as each of the flats became empty, and before they were tenanted again.

'What's going on in number 16?' asked Mrs Peters after she had seen workmen moving into her old home with the tools of their trade, a large aluminium teapot, several chipped mugs, some bags of sugar and packets of tea.

'They're going to do a few alterations before the next tenant moves in,' I said rashly.

'What sort of alterations?' she wanted to know.

I put her into the picture as briefly as I could, but there was a gleam in her eye that worried me.

When the old-fashioned range and the overmantel mirror had been taken away on a junk merchant's lorry, and the new fireplace was in place, the residents began to notice a change coming over Mrs Peters. The breathing that had been such a trial before she moved into Flat 4a began to trouble her again and the legs that had found new strength when the letter arrived to say she could move began to falter when anybody was watching her progress along the verandah. But other than clutching at her blouse and allowing her hand to tremble ever so slightly when I visited her she put on a brave front. Even the workmen were driven to comment on the old lady's indefatigable spirit that triumphed over her frail body. They mentioned it to me when I was sitting on an upturned bucket having a cup of tea with them one morning.

'She's a tough old biddy, and no mistake,' they said admiringly when they were telling me how the tough old biddy had tottered into the stripped-down living room to advise them on the best way to fix the new corner shelves.

'If you don't keep her out of here we'll go on strike,' they said angrily after a week or two of having her as their foreman. But Mrs Peters had no intention of being kept out. She had already formulated her plans for the future and was determined that the structural changes that were being made on the flat she had so recently vacated, and was now so anxious to get back into, were done to her specifications.

She started the wearing-down process on me after the last workman had left, taking with him the aluminium teapot, the mugs, and what was left of the sugar and tea. The tools of the trade had gone before.

'Can you smell gas?' she asked me, after she had rung her bell and got me over before breakfast.

'No,' I said, sniffing hard. 'Why, can you?' She sniffed even harder.

'Indeed I can,' she said. 'It's all over the place. I've hardly had a wink with it. The gas pipes in this flat have never been right since that time when Miss Lilian got blown out of bed. I expected to go up any minute.'

Miss Lilian had never been blown out of bed. The gasmen had called early one morning to make a small adjustment to her cooker and the incident had stuck in her mind. She had become very confused about it until at last she was going around telling everybody that she had been blown out of bed. There was absolutely no foundation whatsoever to the story. But the rumour had spread in the way that rumours do and in the end I stopped bothering to deny them. Miss Lilian occasionally added a little fuel to the fire by telling people that not only was she blown sky high but poor Tommy had needed several stitches to repair the damage done to his tail when he returned to earth.

After I had inhaled deeply again I told Mrs Peters that all I could smell was the aerosol spray she used to counteract other odours. I promised her that in the event of her rising suddenly from her bed one night it would be something less dramatic than a gas leak that had precipitated the move. Then I left her to think up other ways of starting the ball rolling in the direction she wanted it to go.

Her next inspiration came one evening while I was watching 'Coronation Street' and wondering why so many exciting things happened to others and not to me. Hearing her emergency bell I hurried over to find out what had happened to Mrs Peters. I hoped it was nothing too exciting.

'Whatever's the matter with you?' I asked rather crossly when I saw her slumped in a chair with a haunted look in her eyes.

'I've just seen a ghost,' she groaned. I sighed. This was certainly an inspiration.

'There aren't such things,' I said. 'You're imagining it.' I hadn't believed in ghosts since the night I was frightened to death by one at the hospital I was evacuated to while the war was on. Even then it hadn't been a ghost. It had been a life-size plaster cast that was propped up behind a lavatory door and illuminated by the light of the moon streaming through the window. But I had done a lot of screaming before I would believe it wasn't a ghost.

'It was a ghost,' quavered Mrs Peters, in a very old-ladyish quaver. 'I saw it as plain as I'm seeing you. It was that Miss Lilian that used to live here. She was standing at the kitchen door with the ginger cat. She'd got her hat and coat on. I'd have known her anywhere.'

'Well, that's wrong for a start,' I said. 'It couldn't have been Miss Lilian's ghost you saw because she's not even dead. She's still in the hospital up the road and the last time I saw her she was doing fine.' The last time I had seen Miss Lilian she was pacing up and down a long corridor hearing voices in her head and scolding Tommy for not eating the kippers she'd bought for him. The only consolation I had was that she seemed quite happy.

When I went to call on Mrs Peters the following morning she was still in bed. I was rather surprised at this. Usually she was up and about long before the other residents were astir.

'Why are you still in bed?' I asked her, hoping there was a good reason for it.

'It's the ghost,' she said tremulously. 'I've never stopped shaking since I saw it last night.' She shook violently, making the bed move on its castors. 'It gave me such a turn that you'll have to send for the doctor to give me something to settle me down.' She raised her head an inch off the pillow. 'The way I'm going I shan't be here much longer.'

The doctor was a conscientious young man who had only recently arrived, with many other young doctors, from the country of his origin. He had never met Mrs Peters before. He went over her chest, back and front. He tapped her tummy and stroked her big toes. He tenderly felt her glands, looked into her eyes and ears, subjected her tongue to a close scrutiny and gazed long and earnestly down her throat. Then he listened in respectful silence while she told him about the ghost and the effect it had had on her nerves. She would, she said, never be right until she was moved out of the haunted flat, and to the one on the other end of the verandah.

He nodded gravely, patted her hand and told her not to worry, he'd have her better in no time. Then he uncapped his pen and wrote a letter for me to give to the committee and went off as pleased as punch at the way he had coped with his first really difficult case.

When I got back to the patient after seeing the

doctor to his car she was out of bed and putting on her corsets. I handed her the knickers that were draped over a chair and helped her on with her stockings.

'You knew,' I said accusingly. 'You knew all the time that your own doctor was on holiday and it would be his new young locum who would come.' She slipped a petticoat over her head.

'Some of them foreigners aren't bad,' she said, holding up a foot for me to put a shoe on. 'I've nothing against them myself though I can't say I'd have liked a daughter of mine to marry one of them. She'd have had to be shouting at him all the time to make him understand what she was talking about. It's a funny thing about foreigners, they all seem deaf.'

The committee asked a lot of questions when I gave them the doctor's letter. But his word was law. They told me that I must be firm with Mrs Peters and make her understand that this was positively the last time they would let her move from one flat to another. I got the impression that they were holding me responsible for it all.

When I rang Mrs Peters' relations to tell them she was on the move again they didn't seem very surprised. They kindly offered to come and give a hand but I said we could manage nicely, thank you. We had managed without them when they were all at their grandmother's funeral, and we would do so again. I was feeling very huffy at the time.

The vicar popped in to see me one afternoon after he'd been to tea with Mrs Peters in her new flat. He said that she hadn't seemed too happy about things. She missed the range with the mirrored overmantel and didn't care for the colour of the tiles in the new modern fireplace.

'She's quite a character, isn't she?' he said. I had to admit that she was.

Chapter Eleven

IF BRINGING A four-legged friend into the Lodge was forbidden by the charitable body, anybody moving in with a piano was regarded with the greatest disfavour by those already in residence. The committee deliberated for a long time before they consented to such a thing happening. Some of the older members remembered times past when a piano was allowed to cross one of the thresholds and it had caused a lot of unrest. Though the walls of the whitewashed building were thick by modern standards, the sound of a practice run could easily penetrate them unless the soft pedal was put into constant use.

It made little difference to the reluctant audience whether the owner of the piano was a gifted musician, or merely a casual strummer; they were as likely to complain about a classical recital beautifully played as they were to ring their emergency bells when their afternoon nap was disturbed by a spirited rendering of a more popular piece. There was a time and a place for everything, and the middle of the afternoon, just as everybody was settling down for a nap, was no time to be waltzing with Strauss or beer drinking with a lot of students in Heidelberg. Since afternoon naps were a ritual at the Lodge everybody feared the worst when rumours were confirmed that Miss Harrison and her piano were next on the list for admission.

Miss Harrison and her instrument were as inseparable as Miss Lilian and her cat had once been. Those who had known her since her gifted childhood told me that the upright Broadwood had always been something of a mixed blessing. It had stood in the way of her doing a great many things she might have done but for her devotion to it. From the moment she was plonked on a stool and introduced to middle C she had become addicted to it and the other seven notes of the octave almost to the exclusion of all else. She practised her scales when she should have been skipping her days away with playmates, and she dreamed of Chopin instead of mooning over the local boys. In the end it was the piano that put the damper on any hopes she ever had of getting married.

According to hearsay, and I heard a lot of hearsay when I was doing the rounds, the only man to have offered his hand in marriage to Miss Harrison wouldn't have known Chopin from Adam. After it had been wisely decided that such a gap in his education might someday ruin all chance of happiness, Miss Harrison had tearfully returned his ring and the tone-deaf suitor went off to Australia.

Years later there was a grossly exaggerated account of his antipodean adventures in the local paper. The article was headed 'Local Boy Makes Good', and went on to tell the folks back home how the one or two sheep he'd started off with when he first got over there had multiplied until he was now a millionaire. When she had finished reading the article Miss Harrison sat down at her piano and played a few bars of 'Will he no come back again?', then put the past behind her. But there were some around the Lodge who still thought it was a pity that the young man hadn't known as much about music as he seemed to know about sheep. Instead of being a millionaire he could have been happily married to Miss Harrison and they could have played duets together.

The piano was very large. It required four strong men to unload it off the furniture van, and when they had, and had finished examining themselves for ruptures, they spent a long time pushing and shoving it about until they found a suitable place for it in the tiny flat, where it dwarfed everything, even the built-in dresser.

The cottage that Miss Harrison had lived in all her life was due for demolition. It had been due for demolition so long that the piano had sadly deteriorated over the years. Owing to the damp conditions it had lived under, several of its notes no longer responded to pressure, there were unmistakable signs of mildew on the little ruched curtains in the front, and the pair of candlesticks which should have swivelled at a touch were firmly stuck. As well as all this half a leg was missing.

To correct the unsteadiness caused by the loss of half a leg, a large family Bible was wedged under the half that was there. Whenever Miss Harrison wished to consult the Bible on any matter she had to get somebody to steady the piano while she removed the wedge. A fringed silk shawl was draped casually over the lid and there was a rather sad looking aspidistra in the middle.

As well as the aspidistra on the piano there was a glass dome on the dresser. Under the dome were three waxy arum lilies and a ribbon with RIP embroidered on it. The dome was all that was left to remind Miss Harrison of the grave where her parents were laid to rest when they succumbed to influenza during the epidemic after the first war. The cemetery went when a new motorway was planned to run right through it. Miss Harrison rescued the arum lilies before the bulldozers moved in, and resolutely refused to think about the events of one dark night when what was left in the graves was taken to another cemetery on the other side of the town.

It wasn't long before the mournful plaint of Mimi's lover started seeping through the walls of Miss Harrison's flat into those adjoining. The plaint got a mixed reception. One of the adjoining flats was occupied by Mrs Beauchamp, another by Mrs Marsh. They had varying opinions on the Bohemian theme. While Mrs Beauchamp sat on her chaise longue with her eyes closed, swaying dreamily to the tune, Mrs Marsh stomped around her flat, and hammered on the wall, threatening in a loud voice that if the noise didn't cease forthwith (or words to that effect), she would go straight to the charities and get it stopped. She didn't mind a bit of music, she said, she'd always been partial to Gracie Fields, it was this classical stuff that she couldn't stand. She didn't even mind a bit of opera now and again, so long as it was lively. But she drew the line at the ones about people killing themselves or going off their heads. And she couldn't stand the one about that young woman who was supposed to be dying of consumption in an attic. All that rubbish about her hands being cold was a load of codswallop. She knew a lot about consumption, she said, her sister having died of it before she was sixteen. Her sister's hands were never cold, said Mrs Marsh, she'd never known them when they weren't burning hot.

'But that was darling Mimi who was dying in the attic,' said Mrs Beauchamp, opening her eyes and stopping swaying for a moment. 'And the reason her hands were always so cold was because she and some students she was friendly with at the time lived in an attic and they were all too poor to have a fire in the bedroom.'

Mrs Marsh looked very shocked. 'Well, all I can say is, if she'd been a decent sort of girl she wouldn't have been living in an attic with a lot of students. And we could never afford a fire in the bedroom but my sister's hands were still hot. She used to sleep with me and I could feel them burning through my nightdress when she kept me awake with her coughing. She coughed a lot before she died, my sister did.'

Mrs Beauchamp laid her cool hand on her friend's arm and showed by the tears in her eyes how affected she had been by the sad little story.

Since the time that her young man went off to be a millionaire until just before she came to live at the

Lodge, Miss Harrison had been the organist at the church where she had been baptized, and where her parents were married. The church was small, and the organ a simple affair of one keyboard, a few pipes, stops and foot pedals. Originally it had been supplied with air by a boy who sat pumping at the bellows while at the same time reading a comic.

When the organ blower's services were dispensed with and the organ electrified, Miss Harrison found it hard to adjust to the change. Either she attempted to play before the thing was switched on, or she stood on the pedals when it was in full voice. If nothing happened when she sat down to play she got into a fluster looking for the switch. The jumble of noise that arose when she stood on the pedals thinking it was all turned off made her flush with embarrassment.

But from all accounts she had been a very good organist until advancing years, poor eyesight, and even poorer hearing put an end to her regular Sunday employment. Her playing became so erratic that it was often impossible for the congregation to keep up with her or her with them. Often she would cease playing halfway through a hymn, leaving the songsters with their mouths open, waiting for her to start the next verse. Or she went on playing when there were no more verses to sing, and only tailed off gradually after she had looked in the little mirror above the keyboard and seen the vicar discreetly signalling to let her know he was ready to start reading the lesson.

This had been going on for a long time before the parochial church council plucked up courage to pension her off. They did it in easy stages. First, they let her play on alternate Sundays, the vicar making sure that the hymns and psalms he chose were familiar enough for the organist and congregation to finish simultaneously. Then, it was tactfully suggested that she should oblige once a month, then every two months. And finally came the Sunday when she was presented with a small cheque and a zip-up Bible. Nice things were said about her at a do that was held in the parish hall, for which everybody made some sort of contribution in the form of scones, cakes or little savouries.

Thereafter, for as long as she was able to get to church, she sat in a pew close to the altar rails, so that she wouldn't have to walk too far to receive the bread and wine that would sustain her soul for another week. But until the day that she could no longer struggle to church she sank to her knees when prayers were being said. Not for her the bowed head, the eyes shaded by a gloved hand. Down she went on the hassock, her knees cracking like pistol shots. She would have deemed it an insult to her Maker not to have knelt meekly before him while she was acknowledging her manifold sins and wickedness, and admitting that she had erred and strayed like a lost sheep.

All this I heard from the vicar himself. He it was who had exerted pressure on the committee to offer a place in the Lodge for Miss Harrison and her piano. Being a vicar, though now retired and only called upon to officiate when there was a shortage of curates, he still had some pull with the charitable body. He used it to overcome their resistance to the piano.

The vicar told me other things about Miss Harrison. In order to keep her mind even more resolutely off the young man in Australia, she had been the mistress of a small school attended by the daughters of a handful of the better-off tradesmen in the town. Though not quite gentry, they were genteel enough to satisfy the slightly snobbish standards which Miss Harrison set for her school. They could also afford the very small fee she charged for endeavouring to turn their daughters into ladies. Since she spent more time teaching them how to be ladies than she spent on educating them they left her establishment little the wiser than they were when they went there. But since none of them ever expected to have to work for a living the things they had learned were usually enough to keep them sitting prettily until their future fell in their laps.

Miss Harrison wouldn't have approved of her girls working for a living. She might have stretched a point at something like nursing, which she and my mother were convinced was a ladylike occupation, or she might have shown grudging approval of a girl who had decided to become a governess, but only if the children she was to be a governess to were a notch or two higher in the social scale than she was herself. But she would still have preferred her girls to stay at home, balancing books on their heads while their mothers arranged suitable matches. Nobody had arranged a suitable match for Miss Harrison but that hadn't shaken her belief that a woman's place was a step or two behind her husband.

Some of her old pupils used to come and visit her at the Lodge. They were middle-aged, spoke with a genteel accent, and wore gloves and hats. They had been carefully instructed on the proper attire for paying calls. Gloves and hats were obligatory.

But in spite of the rules laid down about the correct way that a lady should dress, Miss Harrison didn't always stick to the rules herself. There were days when she got up in the morning and played her piano instead of putting on her clothes. She was often bare except for a vest when I did the round.

'You'll have to excuse the dishabille, dear,' she would say softly when she opened the door. 'I'm afraid I haven't had time to dress.' Then she would usher me into the piano-filled room.

She was often still in her dishabille, or less, when Dai the Post read out a card that somebody had sent her from the seaside, or when the milkman knocked for his money, or even later when the baker delivered a small white loaf. At first the new butcher boy, who replaced the one that retired, watched eagerly for her bosoms to fall out of her low-cut nightdress, or looked away in embarrassment if she came to the door in her vest. But soon he got bored, and like the others, didn't even notice that she was still in her dishabille.

If it was the vicar that found her in her vest he would shut the door quickly and hurry across to beg me to put her into something more suitable. Then he would hover until I told him it was all right to go in.

The curate who called one day to deliver a marrow and some plaited bread from the harvest festival dropped them on her doorstep and came to tell me they were there. He gave me four King Edward potatoes and a small tin of tomato soup out of the harvest festival gifts as a bribe to say nothing about his cowardice in the face of Miss Harrison's nakedness. The Book of Leviticus was full of warnings about such things, he said.

But however many times I dressed her in something more suitable than a very short vest there was no guarantee that she would stay that way.

'Please, please, dear Miss Harrison,' I said to her once. 'Do try to keep your clothes on while the handyman tacks down the corner of the carpet you tripped over last night.' Tripping over the corners of carpets was something that happened with frightening frequency, together with sliding on slip mats and skidding on polished floors. As fast as I removed a slip mat it was replaced by some houseproud lady, and as often as I pleaded for less polish to be spread on the lino, more was spread when my back was turned. Mirror-bright lino and slippery little slip mats reflected the tender loving care that was taken to ensure that the brittle bones of the elderly were being constantly put at risk.

On the day that I crashed into a cooker after sailing through a living room on a slip mat and sliding through a kitchen on the high-gloss lino, I reinforced the rules about mats that moved and floors that gleamed. But even so there was always the danger of other things happening. Being matron of the Lodge might not have offered much scope for intensive nursing care but it gave me plenty of experience in sitting in waiting rooms until the results of X-rays were known, a diagnosis made and possible admission discussed. I spent many hours in the casualty department comforting old ladies and telling them that it wouldn't be long before they were either at home with something in plaster or lying in a hospital bed with a leg in traction. The wait could be longer if the unfortunate incident had occurred during the weekend, or at some other time when the casualty department was under-staffed, or the radiographers had all gone home.

The handyman's name was Stew. It should have been Stuart but he was slightly ashamed of the fact. He was young and unmarried. I didn't think it was fair that he should get his first good look at the female form while he was tacking down the corner of a carpet. There was always the chance that he would be put off females for ever. There was also the chance that he would be put off music for ever if he came upon Miss Harrison attired only in a vest playing whatever was keeping her glued to the piano that day. It was with these things in mind that I had tried to persuade her to keep her clothes on while Stew was in her room.

But though I had stood over her while she put one garment on after the other, I wasn't surprised when the young man arrived at my door, his face scarlet and his eyes bulging.

'I'm never going in there again,' he gasped, without preamble. 'She was sitting on that piano stool without a stitch on. I didn't know where to look.'

'Don't be silly,' I said sternly. 'Miss Harrison never sits with nothing on, or very rarely. She's almost always wearing a vest.' Even the curate who had brought the marrow and the plaited bread said he thought she might have been wearing a vest.

'Well, all right,' conceded Stew unwillingly. 'Maybe she had got a vest on, but there wasn't much of it and I'm not going in there again, not for you nor nobody else. It isn't decent. My Mum wouldn't like it if she knew.'

I marched him back to Miss Harrison's flat, pushed him through the door and followed him in. Then I stood and held the silk fringed shawl round her frail little body until the last tack was in place. She, meanwhile, giving us a few gems from Gilbert and Sullivan.

'There,' I said to Stew when the job was done. 'There was nothing indecent about that, was there?' He generously admitted that there wasn't.

Being young and adaptable and a willing worker, Stew soon got used to changing light bulbs, putting washers on taps, and fixing fallen curtain rails while

Miss Harrison, dressed or undressed, played a selection of once-popular songs at his special request. I knew that he had come to terms with the rather more mature female form when he stopped me one morning, his face beaming with satisfaction.

'I've put the old girl's leg back on for her so that it doesn't have to have the Bible under it, and I've made a cover for that piano stool of hers, with some foam and a bit of old velvet she'd got. It was enough to give her piles sitting on that horsehair thing with a bare backside. My dad got shocking piles when he was a gravedigger. He said it was with sitting on cold slabs eating his sandwiches. He was always putting ointment on them.' I thanked him for his kindness to Miss Harrison and said that I hoped his dad's piles would improve now that he had retired and no longer had to sit on cold slabs to eat his sandwiches. I also promised to mention the leg and the piano stool when I put in my report to the committee.

Stew started courting soon after that, then he got married. I was pleased about this. It showed that he hadn't been put off the female form by seeing too much of Miss Harrison.

In spite of her habit of taking off her clothes, or not putting them on, Miss Harrison was still able to cope with living in her flat. She was able to cook simple meals when the WRVS ladies didn't come; and with a little encouragement from me she could flick a duster round in between the home-help's visits. It was only after she started confusing night with day that things started getting difficult, and questions were asked about whether she would have to be moved. She answered the questions herself in a most decisive way.

Her neighbours had long ago become reconciled to the stream of melody that assailed their ears during the day. Those who were listening to the wireless or watching television turned up the volume until the strains of 'Clair de Lune' were drowned. The bookworms looked indulgently up from the pages of the latest Barbara Cartland romance they had borrowed from the library, then looked down again, and went back to the make-believe world where all the heroines were perfectly entitled to go to the altar in virginal white.

Even those residents who were trying to have an afternoon nap when Miss Harrison was attempting to get a particularly difficult passage right turned a deaf ear and snuggled down among the pillows.

If anybody happened to hear the piano played when they got up to get themselves a drink in the night, they told themselves that it was perhaps a phase the poor old thing was going through, and given time she would get over it. But things went from bad to worse, until one night Mrs Marsh rang her bell and got me out of bed a couple of hours after I'd got into it.

She was standing in her nighdress glaring at the wall that separated her flat from the one next door.

'Can you hear that?' she said as I walked in. I could. Through the wall came the triumphant crash of a military march played on the loud pedal and with a well-marked beat.

'She's been like that all night,' said Mrs Marsh. 'I haven't been able to shut an eye. You'll have to do something about it or I will.' I stood for a moment admiring the virtuosity of the player, then I went to the flat next door, followed closely by Mrs Marsh, her pigtails sticking out at a jaunty angle. She had no teeth in.

Miss Harrison didn't hear me knocking so I used the master key and went in. Mrs Marsh rushed over to the piano where Miss Harrison was sitting. She was fully dressed and her eyes were closed.

'For Gawd Almighty's sake, do you know what time it is?' Mrs Marsh shouted, slamming down the piano lid and making Miss Harrison move her fingers fast to avoid getting them crushed. She looked first at Mrs Marsh, then at me. She seemed delighted to see us.

'Why, it's the matron and dear Mrs Marsh,' she cried

warmly. 'How nice of you both to come and see me.'

'We ain't come to see you,' shouted Mrs Marsh. 'We've come to tell you to shut your flaming row so that we can all get some sleep. It's nearly two o'clock in the morning, and I haven't closed an eye.' Miss Harrison gave her a sympathetic smile.

'I know exactly how you feel, dear,' she said. 'I had the same trouble myself once.' She turned the sympathetic smile to me. 'And can't you sleep either, dear? You should really do as I did, and go to the doctor. He gave me some pills and told me to take two every night. I still take them and I'm asleep the moment my head touches the pillow.'

I carefully explained that the reason neither Mrs Marsh nor I were asleep was because she had chosen a bad time to play a military march, then I helped her to get undressed, tucked her into bed and went off with Mrs Marsh. We were hardly out of the door before the march tune struck up again. Mrs Marsh clutched her head and groaned.

'That's done it,' she said wildly. 'That's her lot. She'll have to go.'

'But where will she go to?' I asked, after I had put Mrs Marsh's kettle on to make us both a nice cup of tea. I knew there was no place for Miss Harrison to go where she would be as happy as she was at the Lodge.

'She'll have to be put away,' said Mrs Marsh, blowing on her tea. 'She'll have to be sent to that place where Miss Lilian went after she started walking up and down the town with that cat of hers.' I promised that I would do everything in my power to see that she wasn't disturbed again in the night by Miss Harrison and her piano, then I went home.

Already there was a streak of pink in the sky. Soon the dawn chorus would start up and in all too short a time my alarm clock would go off and another day would begin. I went to bed, wondering what I was going to do about Miss Harrison.

But things looked different in the morning. Mrs Marsh wasn't nearly as keen on having Miss Harrison sent away when the sun was shining, and the music that came through her wall was a gentle serenade, only just loud enough to be heard above the ordinary morning sounds.

'I suppose you couldn't have the poor old cow put away just for playing the joanna,' she said, proving that she had a very kind heart under the bib of her faded pinny. 'After all, she doesn't do nobody any harm, and she can still manage to feed herself even if she is off her rocker sometimes. Maybe if I was to take her a nice basin of jellied eels in for her supper she would drop off after she'd eaten them instead of keeping me awake half the night.'

'And, what if she doesn't like jellied eels,' I asked.

Mrs Marsh looked at me in amazement. 'Everybody likes them,' she said.

'And what if she still keeps you awake even after she's eaten them,' I said.

Mrs Marsh grinned. 'Well, if she does she does,' she said, putting a cardigan on to go to the shops. The musquash was back in its mothballs until the summer was over. 'I got used to the bombing in the war, didn't I? Even if I do get nightmares now and again. So I daresay I shall get used to her in the end. But you might try asking her to use the soft pedal a bit more than she does. Maybe that would make a difference.' I said I would bear it in mind.

But when I mentioned using the soft pedal to Miss Harrison she looked round vaguely and didn't seem to understand what I meant. I left her and went to find Stew.

'Couldn't something be done to keep the soft pedal down all the time and to keep the hard one from going down at all?' I asked him. He said he wasn't sure but he'd ask his dad when he went home for dinner. He went round to his mother's for dinner because his new little wife went out to work.

With the aid of a couple of rubber door stoppers and a bit of padding, he fixed both pedals so that neither of them worked, then he rattled off 'Chinese Chopsticks' while I went into Mrs Marsh's to see how it sounded. I could hardly hear a thing.

The old lady had been playing her variations on the soft pedal for several weeks when Mrs Marsh rang her bell.

'What's wrong with you?' I asked, seeing that there was nothing wrong with her.

'It's her next door,' she said. 'She's gone quiet all of a sudden. Listen.' I listened and couldn't hear a sound.

'But you can't hear her now when she plays,' I said.

'You can in the night if you go to the lavatory. It's not loud enough to disturb you when you're in bed but just enough to hear if you have to get up.' There was still no sound from next door.

'Perhaps she's asleep,' I said.

Mrs Marsh shook her head. 'She wasn't asleep five minutes ago,' she said. 'I got up to go to the lavatory and she was playing that thing with all the alleluias in it. The one you get sick to death of hearing on the wireless at Christmas. She'd done one or two of the alleluias, then there was this bit of a bump and it all went quiet. That's when I thought I'd better ring for you.' I was glad she had. I didn't like the sound of a bit of a bump in the middle of the Halleluia Chorus. I went next door with the old, familiar feeling of panic that every nurse gets when she's not sure what awaits her on the other side of a door.

'Poor old girl,' said Mrs Marsh, looking down sadly at Miss Harrison who had slipped off her piano stool, perhaps right in the middle of an alleluia. 'I'm glad we didn't have her put away, aren't you?' I was indeed. I was also glad that she was wearing her best hat and coat when she went. It seemed more in keeping with the grandeur of Handel than a skimpy little vest.

Chapter Twelve

I HAVE ALWAYS liked Christmas. I loved the Christmases of the past, when I was a resident nurse in hospital. I remember wards garlanded with paperchains, paper-petalled lamp shades, and huge trees with very small fairies poised on the top. There was the Mayor, also garlanded with chains, who came to carve the turkeys, and to help us dish out the dinners to patients whose fate it was to have to spend Christmas in hospital. It wasn't too bad a fate, unless the thing that kept them there was too awful for them to enjoy even the thinnest slice of turkey. Rules were relaxed, visitors came and went, and were allowed to sit on the nice clean counterpanes, a crime they were expelled for on less festive occasions. And because it was Christmas even the most niggly ward sister could be found in her office sometime during the great day dispensing small doses of non-medicinal potions which the teetotallers amongst her nurses virtuously declined.

Just as memorable are the Christmases I have spent deceiving my daughters into believing that if they were good little girls, and went to bed early (and didn't get up too early), Santa would nip down the chimney sometime during Christmas Eve, and drop whatever they wanted into the stockings they hung by the fireside. The only stipulation I made, apart from them being good, was that the things they wanted shouldn't be too numerous, or too costly.

Later, when there were grandchildren to deceive, the task was made harder by the installation of central heating. Santa needs chimneys if he is to function properly.

But Christmases at the Lodge were different from any that had gone before. Nobody there believed in Santa Claus; there were no paperchained wards and no towering trees with fairies on the top. There wasn't even a Mayor to come and carve the very small chickens which those who weren't going anywhere usually had for their dinner. But there were plenty of small doses of non-medicinal potions drunk to toast the birth of the Holy Babe. So many, in fact, that unless I said a very firm 'no' to some that were pressed on me when I did the Christmas morning round I could have a little difficulty in locating the latch of my garden gate when the round was over. There are certain risks involved in visiting lonely old ladies on the most important day in the Christian calendar.

Not all the residents were lonely. Most of them had friends and relations, and went off before the fun was due to start and didn't come back until after Boxing Day. Others sat in their best hat and coat and waited to be fetched in time for dinner, and were brought back after the last cracker had been pulled and the final balloon burst.

But neither of these arrangements suited everybody. Mrs Peters declared every year that she would sooner stay at home and eat a chicken leg in peace than have to get dolled up to go to a son or daughter for her dinner.

'But why?' I said, when she told me on her first Christmas at the Lodge that she would rather they forgot all about her and left her in peace. 'I should have thought you'd have been only too happy to be with your family instead of sitting here all by yourself.'

'They'll expect me to give them things,' she said, drawing her mouth down into a bitter line.

'But they'll give you things,' I said. She shook her head.

'Tablets of soap is what I'll get, or another bed jacket, and I've got enough of them to stock a shop with. Nobody ever thinks of giving me a nice set of saucepans which is what I want.'

'But you've got a nice set of saucepans,' I reminded her. 'They clubbed together and bought you a set last year and you've never used them. You're still using the old ones that you've had for so long that the bottoms are nearly dropping out.' She turned on me angrily.

'The reason I've never used them is because they're not the sort I wanted. I wanted copper-bottomed ones, not them flimsy aluminium things what burns the minute you let them boil dry.' I tried to take her mind off unwanted gifts by saying how nice I thought it was of her children to fetch her for dinner on Christmas Day. I didn't say how much I admired them for their courage, though even they never had the courage to extend the invitation far beyond the main midday meal. The very minute the Queen's speech was over they bundled their mother into the car, saying that they thought she should be getting back before it got too dark. They sent her home with mince pies, sausage rolls and rich dark Christmas cake, and even a paper hat and a few crackers so that she could continue the celebrations at home if she felt like it. But she never did. She was always in bed when I popped in to see her later, and the paper hat and crackers were stuffed into the wastepaper basket.

Only once did the Peters family attempt to break the

cords that bound them to her at Christmas and the attempt was doomed before it started.

After they had had a little get-together and decided that just for once, and definitely not to escape from Mother, they would make up a party and go to a hotel for Christmas, leaving Mrs Peters to eat her chicken leg in peace, they came, rather apprehensively, to break the news. She listened to what they had to say, then staggered into the nearest chair, clutching the front of her blouse and vowing that for them to do such an unkind thing would be the death of her. She looked so much as if she was going to die on the spot that they gave her some brandy and loosened her corsets, then sped away to cancel the hotel bookings.

'They didn't want me,' she moaned pitifully when she told me of the dastardly plot to stop her from enjoying her Christmas dinner with her family. 'They only did it because none of them wants to be troubled with me any more. It will be a blessing for all when I'm dead and gone. Maybe then they'll be sorry for the way they treated me when I was here.' I told her not to talk such nonsense, and said how nice it would be for her to have dinner with her family as she had been doing for years. She shook her head.

'It won't be nice at all,' she said. 'I've never been a lover of turkey, and plum pudding repeats on me for days. I'd far rather they left me in peace than dragged me out in the cold just to eat a bit of dinner.' I left her in peace. I was no better at saying the right thing to Mrs Peters than her children were.

In response to the many broad hints I got about the gifts I'd be receiving from the residents, I went out and bought a very small gift for each of them. I made sure that Mrs Peters' name wasn't on one of the tablets of soap I bought in quantity, and since the sum set aside for the annual expenditure didn't run to bed jackets it seemed safe to assume that the lavender bag I gave her one year would be enough of a novelty to please her. It didn't.

'Take it away,' she cried after she had removed the holly-berried wrappings. She gave an explosive sneeze. 'Take it away before it does me a mischief.'

'Whatever's wrong with it?' I asked, half expecting to see a Colorado beetle crawl out of the little lacy bag. She sneezed again.

'It's the lavender. I've got one of them algies to it. Take it away before I have one of my bad attacks.' Since it was unthinkable that she should have one of her bad attacks on Christmas Day of all days, I re-wrapped the little bag and took it away.

I was walking along the verandah, thinking how very much easier it was to offend Mrs Peters than to please her, when her son arrived. I waited until he was almost at her door then went to wish him a Happy Christmas, and also to tell him how I had unwittingly aggravated his mother's 'algie' to lavender. A haunted look came over his face.

'Oh God, now you've done it,' he said despairingly.

'What have I done?' I asked, thinking that all I had done was give his mother yet another unwanted gift.

'You've ruined our Christmas, that's what you've done,' he said. 'She'll be sneezing her head off all day. We had it once before, but it was a clove orange then that somebody gave her and she said she was allergic to.' I said I was sorry for ruining their Christmas, it hadn't been done intentionally and I hoped he'd forgive me. He gave a resigned shrug.

'Oh, forget it,' he said. 'If it hadn't been that it would have been something else. The Christmas before last she flew off the handle because we didn't give her a set of saucepans, last year she flew off the handle because we did. Then there's the dinner. Either there's not enough seasoning in the stuffing or there's too much peel in the pudding. It's the same every year.' I again wished him a Happy Christmas and he went to fetch his mother. I could hear her sneezing at him when I went in to Miss Coombe.

Miss Coombe never went anywhere for Christmas.

She had a cousin who always invited her, and even included the budgerigar in the invitation, but the cousin had a cat, and knowing the things that a cat could do to a budgerigar Miss Coombe declined the invitation with thanks. She was happy to be on her own, she said, with just the dear little budgie for company. I knew this was true. I had proof of it once after she had been prevailed upon to go on an outing to a stately home with one of the women's organizations in the town. She had discussed it at great length with me, begging me to be perfectly honest and tell her if she should go or not. I said I thought she would enjoy it very much and even helped her to choose something suitable to wear. On the morning of the outing she rang her emergency bell to tell me she had a migraine, and asked me to telephone the women's organization to say she wouldn't be going. After a few more migraines nobody invited her anywhere, which suited her very well.

'Good morning, dear, and a Happy Christmas to you,' she said. Billy, who as yet hadn't come to his untimely end, gave a perfect mimicry of the greeting, and I sat down. I gave her my present and she gave me hers, which proved to be a straight exchange, then she did as she always did on Christmas morning.

'Perhaps you would care to join me in a small glass

of sherry,' she said, indicating the bottle and two glasses on the table. 'I assure you that it is British and very sweet. I am sure that one small glass couldn't possibly do you any harm.' I said that I would be delighted to join her in a small glass of sherry. After I had drunk it and scratched the budgie under the chin I went on my way. I knew from the smell of roasting coming from the kitchen that she would be enjoying a Christmassy sort of dinner, even if she was eating it alone, except for the budgie of course.

The sherry I drank with Miss Macintosh was neither British nor over-sweet. Nor was it in a very small glass. She offered me a nip of something stronger first, but I declined it, saying that I had never acquired a taste for her native brew. She said that though she didn't make a habit of indulging she hardly thought the charitable body would object to a little relaxing of the rules on Christmas Day. I said something about what the eye didn't see the heart wouldn't grieve over and we both laughed merrily over the little joke. I always laughed a lot when I visited Miss Macintosh on Christmas morning. By the time I got round to Mrs Turgoose I was ready to laugh at anything.

Mrs Turgoose went out every year for her Christmas dinner. She sat in her hat and coat waiting for a volunteer from one of the churches or chapels to come and collect her to spend the day with them. The invitation was one she had angled for long before Christmas.

The only time Mrs Turgoose went to church or chapel was on the Sunday when names were being taken of those who wished to be invited out for Christmas Day, and those who wished to receive a hamper when the harvest festival gifts were being distributed. As she would have been the first to admit, she was never backward in coming forward when there was a chance of getting something for nothing.

In the short space between me walking in and the church or chapel volunteer arriving there was usually time for at least one glass of sherry and two or three little anecdotes accompanied by much nudging and winking. Mellowed by all the glasses I raised to toast the Babe I sometimes even added an anecdote or two of my own, upon which Mrs Turgoose nudged me even harder and I gave her a dig in retaliation.

Miss May was usually the last to offer me a tiny drop of something which she kept on the dresser in case of emergencies. She also was on the list of eligibles for an invitation for Christmas dinner, not because she had made it her business to be present when the list was drawn up, but because she kept in regular contact with the Methodist Church and the C of E. She kept in regular contact with the RCs as well, but her conscience never allowed her to accept any of their invitations.

Preparing Miss May to go out for dinner took up quite a lot of time. She had to be wrapped in enough shawls to make her impervious to the least puff of wind. She caught cold easily and Miss May with a cold could lessen the chance of a Happy New Year for me – or at least of a Happy New Year's Eve.

Because she was a very nervous lady great care had to be taken when loading her into the car. First she had to be assured that whoever was driving it knew how to drive. Then rugs had to be tucked in on all sides of her knees, an extra shawl fetched and a warmer pair of gloves found, but at last she was off and I felt free to go home where my own family was waiting for me. Somebody gave me a hair of the dog that had bitten me ever so slightly, then we got on with our own Christmas, happy in the knowledge that all was well with the Lodge and nobody was without some sort of reminder that it was a very special day.

But however muddled my head may have been when I had finished the Christmas morning round none of it could be blamed on Mrs Marsh or her bosom friend. From the first Christmas that Mrs Beauchamp came to live at the Lodge it had been an understood thing that her son would invite Mrs

Marsh to share their turkey on Christmas Day, and Mrs Marsh's son would invite Mrs Beauchamp on Boxing Day.

The arrangement had bothered me when I first heard that it was under discussion. I had visions of Mrs Marsh shocking the upper-crust company she would be eating her dinner with by passing on some of the jokes which her husband had passed on to her when he was a humper in Smithfield. I feared what their reaction would be if she went into detail about the things that might have happened to Evelyn if he had become a humper instead of a City gent.

I also wondered what would be Mrs Marsh's son's reaction if Mrs Beauchamp had one of her little lapses and mistook him for the butler when he was handing her a plate of chicken. They would be having chicken on Boxing Day, Mrs Marsh told me, because her son reared them in his backyard and since they would be having turkey at Mrs Beauchamp's son's place they wouldn't want it twice on the trot. Having it twice on the trot might give them the trots, she said, waiting for the feeble joke to get a laugh. I smiled politely.

But I needn't have worried about the success of the arrangement. According to the things they told me after Christmas it had gone like a bomb.

'Such a splendid example of the British working

man,' breathed Mrs Beauchamp of Mrs Marsh's son. 'He put me in mind of one of the under-gardeners we used to have at the Manor. Nanny always made me look the other way when we came upon him in the grounds. He never seemed able to button up the front of his trousers properly. I noticed that dear Mrs Marsh's son seemed to have the same problem, especially after he had eaten his dinner. Though I looked away of course, it made me feel quite at home.'

'That Evelyn of hers wasn't half as stuck up as I'd expected him to be,' said Mrs Marsh when she was giving me an account of how the monied class spent Christmas. 'He was a bit offhand with me when we first got there but he loosened up a lot after he'd had something out of one of them bottles they had on the dresser. Real cut glass they were by the looks of them.'

'What happened after he'd loosened up?' I asked her.

'He carved the turkey and he gave us one lot of wine to drink with that and another sort to have with the pudding. I'm not all that fond of wine so I asked him if he happened to have any Guinness in the house, and it turned out that he had. When we'd eaten the pudding which was a bit too rich for my liking they put some cheese on the table, but it had gone a bit mouldy so I didn't have any. I was full up anyway. They had cups of coffee but I told them it didn't agree with me so they made me a nice cup of tea instead. After that I came over a bit sleepy so I put me feet up on the couch and had forty winks. I must say they made me very welcome but I couldn't help laughing when anybody called him Evelyn.'

Mrs Marsh had obviously enjoyed rubbing shoulders with the rich as much as Mrs Beauchamp had liked hobnobbing with the lower classes.

Chapter Thirteen

WE WERE OFTEN well into January before the post-Christmas aches and pains, little tummy upsets, and other things brought on by the annual orgy were starting to improve. But then came the worst of the weather and there were more serious things to trouble us. The slippery pavements made shopping dangerous, and even those who liked to get out were put off by the bitter winds. Some simply hibernated with coughs, colds and wheezy chests, while others disobeyed their doctors and sat round the fire when he had told them to stay in bed.

Miss May caught a chill every winter and frightened herself, and everybody else, into thinking she wouldn't live to see another spring. Her little bamboo bedside table was so stacked with bottles of medicine, pots of embrocation and boxes of pills and tablets that there was no room left for the lemon and barley water, tins of mint humbugs and assortment of biscuits that she needed to stay her between the boiled egg she had for breakfast and the fillet of plaice she picked at for lunch.

Several times a day she covered her head with a towel and brought it out beaded with moisture from the medicated steam she inhaled from a jug. Several times a day she turned this way and that while I rubbed her chest with camphorated oil and applied wintergreen lotion to her aching joints. I was always greatly relieved when Miss May took her first tottering steps across the room. It was as sure a sign that spring was on the way as the first crocus.

There were other complaints that kept me more than usually busy during a winter that started early and finished late. For want of a better name the complaints were being called viruses. Having a virus became almost a status symbol at the Lodge. Even Miss Coombe's new little budgie got one. But the vet managed to pull him round.

When Mrs Beauchamp was told by her doctor that she'd got a virus, Mrs Marsh became almost as ill as her friend.

'Will she get over it?' she asked me a dozen times a day. I had nursed so many viruses since the winter started that I knew, given the proper course of antibiotics, the one that Mrs Beauchamp had would respond well to treatment and be gone quite soon. But nothing I said would convince Mrs Marsh. Having a virus was a different matter altogether from having something as ordinary as double pneumonia or pleurisy. There was a sinister ring about the obscure term which frightened Mrs Marsh. Though she wouldn't have wanted Mrs Beauchamp to have either double pneumonia or pleurisy, she could have coped with them better than she could cope with a virus. She wandered up and down the verandah waiting for the doctor to leave the sick room, and looked into his face for signs that she would soon be having to borrow black for the funeral. His face told her nothing. He was a cheerful young man who always managed to look hopeful even when there was little hope.

But the antibiotics worked their miracles and it wasn't long before Mrs Beauchamp was well enough to go to bingo if it was neither snowing nor raining on Wednesday afternoon. Mrs Marsh was quite proud of her for having a virus. She boasted about it during the interval between sessions.

'She was practically at death's door,' she told everybody who would listen. 'She had one of them whatsits that everybody seems to be getting these days. It's a wonder she's here to tell the tale.' Mrs Beauchamp fluttered her lashes modestly.

After Miss May, Mrs Beauchamp and Miss Coombe's budgerigar had recovered from their own particular whatsit, and spring seemed just around the corner, there was an event that brought a little excitement to banish the blues of winter. An invitation arrived from an exclusively male and Very Important Lodge in the town, requesting the pleasure of the company of the residents of our not nearly so important Lodge at a dinner to be given them as a belated Christmas present. Each of the ladies received a card, gold embossed and very posh. I got one as well.

The cards were simply worded, giving place, date and time, and expressing the wish that all who intended availing themselves of the invitation should put a 'yes' on the line marked with a cross and return the card in the stamped addressed envelope enclosed therewith. Those who didn't intend going for any reason were asked to put a 'no'. It was all perfectly clear. There was nothing on the card that anybody could possibly have misunderstood, or not have understood. Yet I knew as I read it that the rounds I did that day would take longer than usual.

I had been at the Lodge long enough to know that not everybody would grab a pen and write a breathless 'yes' on the line marked with a cross. There would be those who would look at the card, turn it over and examine it from every angle, read the words, puzzle over them, worry over them, then wait for me to explain what it was all about. Even then they would puzzle and worry for another few days before they committed themselves to anything.

Others would rack their brains to think up reasons for refusing the invitation as they had refused all other invitations to similar functions. They would plead that they were shy amongst strangers, and especially among strange men; they didn't like going out at night; and, as a last resort, their absolute certainty that they would be feeling far from all right on the night.

Those who put patches on their pinny would say they hadn't a thing to wear, and those who didn't put patches on anything wouldn't have a rag to wear either. It would be my responsibility to overcome all these objections, and get as many acceptances as possible on the line marked with a cross. I foresaw trouble ahead. I began the assault course with Mrs Peters.

She was standing on the hearthrug holding the card at arm's length between thumb and finger. She looked as if she was as allergic to it as she had been to the lavender.

'And what's this supposed to mean?' she asked in her most truculent voice. I took the card from her and examined it closely.

'It's an invitation from the Masons to go to a Christmas dinner,' I answered, hoping to have solved the problem in one illuminating sentence. Mrs Peters snatched the card off me.

'I know it's an invitation to a Christmas dinner,' she said, in a voice of disgust. 'I may be old but I'm not stupid. I can read, you know.' I apologized for anything I might have said to imply either that she was stupid or couldn't read, and asked her what there was about the card that she didn't understand.

'There's nothing about it that I don't understand. What I don't understand is what it's all about. Men like them on this card don't ask the likes of us for Christmas dinner without a good reason, especially when it's nearly Easter. I should want to know what the reason was before I said I'd go, and then there'd be no guarantee that I'd go. You mark my words, there's more behind this than meets the eye.'

'They're just being kind,' I said. 'And what could there possibly be behind some nice gentlemen like the Masons inviting a few elderly ladies out for the evening?' Mrs Peters gave me a look that was full of hidden meaning.

'Well, we shall see,' she said, leaving a lot of unanswered questions in the air. She scrutinized the card as if searching for the key that might unlock the mystery.

I glanced at my watch and saw that it was time for me to be getting on with the round. Slowly I walked towards the door. Then I played my ace.

'Well, I shouldn't worry about it if I were you,' I said, in a syrupy soothing voice. 'Nobody can make you go anywhere that you don't want to. All you have to do is put a "no" instead of a "yes" and I'll post it when I post the others.' She rose to the bait as I had known she would. I had learned a lot about old lady psychology since I went to work at the Lodge, most of it from little encounters I'd had with Mrs Peters.

'Of course I shall go,' she said indignantly. 'I've got as much right to go as anybody else round here. More than most. I'm one of the oldest residents and don't you forget it.' I handed her my pen and she sat down and wrote a nice big 'yes' on the RSVP line. I put the card into the stamped addressed envelope and congratulated myself on the ease by which I had won the first round.

Miss Macintosh had solved her own problems. All that was worrying her was what she was going to wear on the big night. I promised her that I would go through her wardrobe with her one evening and added her stamped addressed envelope to Mrs Peters'.

Mrs Marsh was already in Mrs Beauchamp's flat when I got there. Laid out on the table was a large selection of gaudy jewellery. Laid out on the bed was a large selection of floor-length gowns, a couple of fur stoles, one or two capes and several evening shawls. The smell of mothballs was overpowering.

Mrs Marsh had on a deep purple georgette gown over her pinny, a tiara-like edifice on her head, a high pearl choker round her scraggy neck, several glittering rings on her fingers and clanking bangles on her wrists. The toes of the slashed-up canvas shoes peeped coyly from beneath the trailing gown.

'Isn't it all too terribly exciting, dear?' said Mrs Beauchamp, waltzing round the room in a flapperish gauzy creation that barely came to her knees. 'But really you know, it's been so long since I was asked out for dinner that I simply cannot make up my mind what to wear. And neither can dear Mrs Marsh.'

Dear Mrs Marsh gave her tiara a twirl. It looked no better the right way round than it had looked when it was back to front.

'It's not bad, is it, mate,' she said to me, simpering at herself in the mirrored door of Mrs Beauchamp's wardrobe. 'I've always fancied myself in a tiara. It makes you feel like a queen with one of these on your head.' The thought flashed through my mind that the selection committee had known what they were doing when they looked elsewhere for their Dowager Queen.

Mrs Marsh didn't look right in a tiara and neither did she suit a floor-length gown. The clothes she always wore were more to her style.

After we had selected and rejected several outfits for Mrs Beauchamp to wear we finally settled for an oyster satin ensemble she had worn when she was presented to one of the minor royalties at a charity bazaar in the days when she was picnicking in the copper belt with Mr Beauchamp, a handful of servants and Apples. It fitted her perfectly. The hunks of buttery French bread she ate with her morning coffee hadn't added an inch to her waistline.

'You'll catch your death in that thing if it's cold when we go,' said Mrs Marsh. 'You'll need something warm round your shoulders, a cardigan or something.'

'But I shall wear my mink cape, dear, and plenty of warm things underneath,' replied Mrs Beauchamp, 'and you can borrow one of the stoles.'

Kitting out Mrs Marsh wasn't easy. We spent a long time robing and disrobing her.

'You really should wear some sort of foundation garment, dear,' said Mrs Beauchamp, casting a critical eye on the lumpiness of the rose-pink confection we had managed, with a great deal of difficulty, to squeeze her friend into. Mrs Marsh shook her head.

'You're not getting me into no armour plate,' she

said roundly. 'I'd be doubled up with heartburn if I was trussed up like that. If I go at all I'll go as nature intended me to be and not done up so that I can't breathe.'

I left them in the middle of a heated discussion about whether the rose pink or the deep purple would do the most for Mrs Marsh. But before I went there was one small thing I had to know.

'How did you come to buy dresses as large as those?' I asked Mrs Beauchamp, looking from her slim figure to the ample gowns.

She gave an embarrassed little laugh. 'I bought them for wearing at functions when I was expecting darling Evelyn. They were a bit on the big side even then but they quite disguised the interesting condition I was in.' She paused for a moment, dwelling on the past. 'You see, my dear, a lady didn't advertise things like that in those days. It quite shocks me to see pictures in the papers of young women bulging out everywhere. I do feel a little modesty is called for in certain circumstances.' I was glad that Mrs Beauchamp took *The Times*. There were pictures in some of the less weighty papers of young women bulging out in a way that would have stunned her.

Miss Coombe was sitting in her rocking chair nervously twisting the gilt-edged card. It was beginning to show signs of wear and tear from being nervously twisted since it was dropped on her mat. The new little budgie that had replaced the one that was eaten was fluttering round his cage making shrill noises. There was seed scattered down on the carpet, and water dripping from the pot he had overturned in his frenzy. He apparently sensed something in the air that unsettled him. He was like a bird demented.

Miss Coombe didn't even bid me good morning when I walked in, and she gave me no time to ask how she was.

'I think there must have been some mistake,' she said, showing me the card. 'The postman delivered this to me this morning and it can't possibly be for me.' I carefully examined the card. It had two tea stains and a blob of marmalade on it which told me that it had arrived while Miss Coombe was having her breakfast. I could imagine her trembling fingers slopping the tea and allowing the marmalade to go astray in her agitation.

I explained as well as I could that all the residents had received a similar card that morning and, if it was any comfort to her, so had I. She seemed no happier after I had finished explaining.

'But I still don't understand,' she said, getting up from her chair and going across to put a soothing finger into the budgie's cage. He responded by taking a vicious peck at it. His name was Joey and he was fast becoming as bad tempered as Billy had been. He was already learning simple phrases like 'Give us a kiss' and 'Who's a pretty boy then?' The time wasn't far away when I would be standing on the sidelines cheering and clapping while he trundled his little celluloid ball between two tiny goal posts.

Miss Coombe left Joey to his own devices and came back to her chair.

'But I still can't imagine why I should have received a card,' she said. 'I don't know any of the gentlemen who belong to this particular Lodge and as far as I can recall none of them know me. I had a cousin once whom we suspected of having some allegiance to the Brotherhood but he never spoke about it to anybody. I'm quite sure the invitation couldn't have come from him.'

I explained again that everybody had had an invitation. It was just a kind thought on the part of the Brotherhood and I hoped she would look upon it as such and put a 'yes' on the dotted line. I saw by her face that she still wasn't convinced. She got up from her chair again.

'I shall have to ask Joey what he thinks before I decide anything,' she said, going across to the cage. She stood for a moment crooning softly to the little bird and he hurled himself from his perch, hung with one claw from his plastic ladder and pecked savagely at his identical twin in the mirror that dangled from the roof of the cage.

'I really believe he is trying to tell me that he doesn't wish me to go,' said Miss Coombe, offering a finger to be jabbed at again. Joey screeched round the cage in a fit of dementia, then went back to attacking his image.

'I think you should go even if he doesn't want you to,' I said. 'You don't go out much and it would make a change for you. And you could wear the nice red dress you always wear at Christmas, and maybe if you put a cover over his cage Joey won't even know that you've gone.' Miss Coombe brightened up for a moment then sank back into gloom.

'I don't know,' she said. 'I've always kept myself to myself and have never been a good mixer. I'm afraid I should feel very out of place on an occasion like this.' I left her to sort it out with Joey.

Mrs Turgoose needed no help from me or anybody else to make up her mind. She was already sitting letting out tucks in the dress she had worn when the Labour Party won the election a month or two before the Second World War ended. It was not only much too tight for her but much too short. I advised her to give it to the next Labour Party Jumble Sale and wear her pinafore dress with a nice blouse under it.

'It'll be quite like old times, won't it?' she said, after she had put the pins away and bundled the dress into a carrier bag with some other things which she was donating to swell the Labour Party funds. 'There's bound to be a drop of gin and a bit of a singsong after we've had our dinner.' I warned her not to bank on it. I said that the gentlemen who'd sent the invitations might not approve of elderly ladies drinking gin. There would perhaps be a couple of 'Auld Lang Synes' and even a short burst of 'For He's a Jolly Good Fellow', followed by the National Anthem, but I thought the chances of any sort of knees-up were very slim. Her face fell.

'Never mind,' I said, trying to cheer her up again. 'There's almost sure to be a glass of sherry, and maybe a drop of non-alcoholic wine to wash the turkey down.' She said she wouldn't say no to the sherry but she hadn't touched non-alcoholic wine since somebody gave her a bottle of it for her nerves when she was on the change and it had tasted of nothing but Oxo. I left her thinking of the days of old when things were done differently.

Miss May had read her card and clearly understood it. But as she said, it was far too soon to say yes or no.

She could be queer again by then, or even dead. You could be here today and gone tomorrow just like Cousin Sid was, so there was no point in looking that far ahead. I said that I entirely agreed, but I still thought she should say yes to the invitation, just in case she was still with us and not feeling queer.

At the end of the day the poll predicted that half the residents would be accepting the invitation, a quarter wouldn't and the rest were doubtful. But by the end of the week I had stuck down all the envelopes knowing that barring accidents, Miss May coming over queer (or worse), or a virus striking, we would be taking our places at the table at the appointed time, and in full strength.

Chapter Fourteen

WHEN THE GREAT day dawned and I opened my curtains and saw the rain falling and the wind blowing through the winter-bare trees, I feared the worst. I knew that however many shawls I wrapped her in it wouldn't be easy to persuade Miss May to leave her nice warm fire, and I was sure that Miss Coombe would use the weather as an excuse to stay at home with Joey. Mrs Marsh would certainly think twice about turning out on a dark and stormy night, and if she started to get obstinate then so would her bosom friend. I put in a quick petition to whoever was responsible for the weather. I wanted us to get to our destination dry, even if we weren't too warm. As well as being wet and windy it was very cold.

It had been very cold since the humid Christmas when the pessimists predicted that the unseasonal weather would be the death of a lot of old people who needed plenty of good sharp frosts to kill the germs before the germs killed them. When the sharp frosts came the pessimists predicted that they would be the death of a lot of old people who didn't have the stamina to stand up to the arctic conditions. I had been a nurse long enough to know that at any given time there would be some old people that would die, and some that wouldn't, whatever the weather.

But the worst of the winter was over. Already the snowdrops were dying off and clusters of crocuses were springing up in the most surprising places. I knew that very soon, if an emergency bell rang at dawn, I would hurry down the path and be filled with content at the signs of spring around me. There would be the crunch of snail shells under my feet and fresh green weeds springing up in the beds where the pansies were still asleep. Later, the blackbird that sang on my television aerial throughout the summer would sing again, and the whole annual rebirth would start again. Even the worst of winters had its compensations.

Because it was the Big Day, the day that had occupied our thoughts since the invitations were received, the first round I did went on for a very long time. I drank endless cups of tea and coffee while I listened to accounts of things that had come on in the night, making it quite impossible for those who had been afflicted to think of going out. I dismissed so many blinding headaches, stabbing pains everywhere and other vague symptoms of imagined illness as feeble excuses that if the Lodge had become rampant with bubonic plague I would have dismissed it just as lightly.

Ladies who hadn't wanted to accept the invitation in the first place, but were talked by me into putting a 'yes', had to be talked again into believing that they had done the right thing, and some who had eagerly penned their acceptance were searching for reasons to go back on their word.

Miss May told me that she had come over ever so queer in the night, and though she had fought to keep her finger off the emergency bell she thought it would be unwise to set foot outside until she had been under the doctor for a day or two. But after I had made her a cup of cocoa and given her two digestive biscuits she rallied enough to show me the blouse and skirt she intended to wear if she was spared.

When I got to Miss Coombe she was having such a terrible attack of nerves that I almost weakened and told her she could stay at home if she wished. Then I had a better idea. I said that though it wasn't Christmas, and still rather early in the morning, we would both have a small glass of sherry to settle her nerves. The sherry must have settled Joey's nerves as well, as he allowed me to stroke his downy breast while he looked complacently at his mate in the mirror.

It was Mrs James, who hadn't been at the Lodge very long and lived below Miss Coombe, who gave me my first real problem. When I knocked at her door she kept me waiting for a minute or two before she opened it the merest crack.

'Oh, it's you,' she said, sounding very relieved. 'I thought it might have been the milkman knocking for his money. Please come in.' I squeezed through the door and came face to face with Mrs James.

'Oh,' I said, putting as little expression as possible into the very small word. 'I see you have had your hair done for tonight.' Mrs James's hair, which was normally a mixture of grey, white and faded mouse, was now a very bright blue. And instead of the smooth neat style I was used to seeing there were hundreds of tight little curls springing up from her scalp.

'Do you think it looks all right?' she asked, anxiously scanning my face, and running her fingers through the azure mop. I made a sound that might have meant anything.

'I've been a bit worried about it since I got up,' went on Mrs James. 'I did it myself last night but the perm seems to have gone a bit tight and I was a bit heavy handed with the blue rinse. I was glad it was you at the door and not the milkman. I was afraid he might have laughed at me.' I knew our milkman. He was far too kind to do anything so brutal. He was the young man with 'Cut Here' tattooed round his neck, and was a great favourite with all his customers. He gave everybody the right change and never charged for pints they didn't have. He would have taken one look at Mrs James's vivid new hair style, then he would have told her what a smasher she was and she'd better watch out or she'd be getting took advantage of. When he brought me my milk he would have mentioned the colour, asked me if it was anything catching, then we might both have laughed, but at the milkman's joke, not at Mrs James.

It took three washes before the azure crown of glory had faded to a washed out palish blue, and by then the tight little curls were so tight that we couldn't get a brush through them; they had to be left looking like wire wool. I told Mrs James that it looked quite nice, which was the kindest thing I could say, then I left her and got on with the round.

As the day wore on the tension spread. No sooner had I left one flat, after assuring whoever lived there that there was nothing at all for her to worry about, than I was in another uttering the same reassurances. Even Miss Macintosh wasn't her usual calm self. She looked very harassed when she opened her door.

'I don't think I shall be going after all,' she said, ushering me into the room. I removed a few garments from one of the chairs and sat down. There were garments on other chairs that looked as if they had been tried on, taken off and tried on again before being thrown off in a final gesture of despair.

'Why ever not?' I asked her.

'I've got nothing to wear,' she said, sounding very low. I knew the feeling. The chairs in my bedroom at home, as well as the floor, not to mention the bed, were strewn with garments I had tried on and taken off in a hurry after I had seen myself in the mirror. Though I went on a different diet nearly every day, the pounds crept up on me. I was still trying to lose the stone I had gained over Christmas.

'Of course you've got something to wear,' I told Miss Macintosh with all the matronly authority that I could muster. 'You've got that nice tartan skirt you wear on Sundays, and the jumper and cardigan you always wear with it.'

'They're past their best,' she said. 'And besides, the others will no doubt be going in long dresses and high-heeled shoes.' She held up a pair of low-heeled sensible brogues for my inspection. They were as past their best as the skirt and twinset were. The regular application of polish, followed by a brisk rub with a soft clean cloth hadn't been enough to arrest their final disintegration. The soles were showing signs of beginning to part from the uppers.

I said that as far as I knew most of her neighbours would be going in the clothes they wore for best, and nothing would induce Mrs Marsh to wear any other shoes than the ones she wore all the time. She wouldn't risk ruining the evening with a pair that hadn't grown accustomed to her feet.

'What's this?' I asked, diving into Miss Macintosh's wardrobe and bringing out a floral dress and jacket that I had never seen her wearing.

'It's a wee thing I bought for the party they gave me when I retired,' she said. 'I've never worn it since. It must have got the moth in it by now.' We examined it carefully. Not surprisingly, since Miss Macintosh had been retired for fifteen years, the voracious little clothes-eater had made many a meal out of the floral material.

'What shoes did you wear with it?' I asked, after I had bitten off the thread from the final hasty repair job.

'I wore these,' she said, looking at the sensible brogues that were much too sensible for the flowery dress and jacket. Suddenly she got a chair and reached to the top of the wardrobe. She took down a cardboard box and apologized for the film of dust that covered it.

She untied the string that was keeping the box together and took out a handful of tissue paper which had gone brown round the edges. Amongst the tissue paper, and stuffed with more of it, was a pair of shoes and a tiny bag. The shoes had spiky heels that were no more than an inch high. The fronts were prettily trimmed with velvet butterfly bows studded with little blue beads.

'But they're lovely,' I said, and meant it. Miss Macintosh took off the very basic slippers she was wearing and put on the spiky-heeled shoes. Even with the thick woollen stockings she had on they still looked pretty.

'I've only worn them once,' she said, rather shyly. 'I bought them years ago when a young man invited me to a dance.' I pricked up my ears, hoping for a story of unrequited love, or a tragic end to a true romance. The fact that Miss Macintosh was unmarried pointed to one or the other. She destroyed the picture with her next words.

'It was his engagement dance and I would never have been invited if the girl he was engaged to hadn't been my best friend at school. I sat with a lot of other girls who had been her best friends and nobody asked us to dance. We ate the refreshments and watched the others dancing. We were what were known as wall-flowers in those days.'

I told her that I knew how it felt to be a wallflower. I had often been one myself at the hospital dances when I was doing my training. I remembered how painful it had been to watch others waltzing and foxtrotting while I ploughed through plates full of sausage rolls and drank pints of lemonade. Then I went off to see how Mrs Marsh and Mrs Beauchamp were getting on.

After a lot of gentle persuasion Mrs Marsh had at last gone to the Co-op and bought herself a corset. She was being ungently forced into it when I arrived on the scene.

'She'll die,' I said warningly, watching her face gradually turning purple. Mrs Beauchamp let go of the back laces and peered round at her friend.

'Of course she won't die,' she said impatiently. 'All she has to do is hold her breath for a few minutes while I finish lacing up the back then everything will be perfectly all right.' She seized the laces in both hands and pulled. There was a rending sound and three hooks detached themselves from the rigid busk front of the corset. Mrs Marsh released her pent-up breath and flopped into a chair.

'Thank Gawd for that,' she said, giving the pound or two of flesh that had escaped from its temporary confinement a good scratch. 'Another minute of that and it would have been curtains for me.'

'Don't talk such nonsense,' said Mrs Beauchamp sternly. 'If you had only done as I asked you and held your breath for a moment or two longer we would have got most of your stomach into the corset. As it is it will bulge out everywhere and ruin the line of your dress.' Mrs Marsh stopped scratching her superfluous flesh and turned on her friend, her bosoms quivering with rage beneath her vest.

'I don't see how it can bulge out any further than yours did when you were expecting your precious Evelyn,' she said furiously. 'And if you think I'm going to strangle meself in one of them things you've got another think coming.' She kicked the corset across the room. 'And what's more, I've half a mind not to go to the flaming dinner. After the way you've been pulling me about I shan't be in any fit state to go.' At this Mrs Beauchamp burst into tears.

'But of course you must go to the dinner,' she said, looking pleadingly at her friend. 'You know perfectly well that Mr Beauchamp has another engagement tonight and I couldn't possibly go to the Embassy without an escort.' Mrs Marsh raised her eyes and touched her temple.

'Gawd, she's off,' she said, picking up the corset and stuffing it behind a cushion.

After she had dressed herself she put an arm round

Mrs Beauchamp. 'All right then, I'll go, so stop carrying on. But like it or lump it, I'm not wearing corsets. If I bulge I bulge, and them as don't like it know what they can do.'

'Yes, dear,' said Mrs Beauchamp meekly.

Mercifully it had stopped raining when the time came for me and a few willing helpers to get the residents onto the forecourt, and into the minibus that had been sent to fetch them. There was almost a full moon to light our way, and a few stars to lend enchantment to the evening. But it was still cold, and most of us wore coats, which rather spoilt the effect of the fineries beneath. I shivered in a little black dress that wasn't very little but was still a size too small for me, and teetered dangerously on heels that were an inch or two higher than the ones I usually wore. The added height caused me to put a hand out to steady myself while I was shepherding the ladies along the verandah, which encouraged a few facetious remarks about the matron's drinking habits. I didn't mind the remarks. I knew that those who were making them were in good spirits and thoroughly looking forward to the evening that lay ahead. There was one who wasn't.

When I went to offer Miss Coombe my arm she hung back nervously and said she was having second thoughts about going out. I reminded her that she had already had second thoughts, and third ones as well, then I eased her into her coat and out of the door. She was reluctant about letting me lock it behind us, and made me go back several times before we got to the end of the verandah, to make absolutely certain that there were no cries of distress coming from the deserted Joey. Instead of being pleased when I told her there wasn't a cheep out of him, she insisted on unlocking the door again so that she could look under the cover of his cage and satisfy herself that he hadn't hanged himself from his little rope ladder or drowned himself in his little pot of water or choked on a millet seed. Once inside her flat she would have taken off her coat and refused to go out again if I hadn't been more than usually firm and said how rude it would be not to go to the dinner after she had put a 'yes' on the card, and when a place would have been laid for her at the table. Even after I had finally got her into the minibus she was still protesting that she had only said she would go because I had bludgeoned her into it. She sat with a rug round her knees, straining her ears for the sound of a little bird eating his heart out.

All the efforts that had been put into the preparations were well worth while. Mrs James had a chiffon scarf over her head. The effect was very pretty. I noticed that she kept the scarf on all the evening but whether because of the wire wool underneath, or because she still wasn't happy about her pale blue hair, I wasn't sure.

Miss Macintosh wore the butterfly-bowed shoes, and carried the matching bag over her arm exactly like the Queen. She had arranged a diamante cluster over the worst of the moth-eaten bodice of the dress and nobody could possibly have guessed that it was as old as it was.

Even Mrs Peters had submitted to a little beauty treatment – albeit ungraciously. One of her daughters had popped in that morning on her way to work and washed and set her hair for her, and another daughter had popped in at teatime on her way from work and put a dab of powder on her mother's nose and a touch of colour on her cheeks. Both daughters had gone home smarting from the things she had said to them in return for their kindness, but Mrs Peters looked prettier than I had ever seen her look, and softer.

Fortunately Miss May had been spared to wear the blouse and skirt she had shown me that morning. When I went to wheel her to the minibus in her mobile chair she was sitting sipping a spoonful of brandy mixed with hot water and sugar. This, she explained, was to ensure that she didn't come over queer before we got to where we were going. She had a black velvet ribbon threaded through her plaits and another round her graceful neck. Somewhere among the lavender bags in one of her drawers she had found a lacy, gossamer shawl which she had crocheted for one of her birthdays before her eyes were weakened with cataracts. I told her how glad I was that she felt able to go, after all the little set-backs she'd been having lately, then I arranged several more shawls over the gossamer one and pushed her across the forecourt.

Mrs Marsh wasn't wearing a coat over the purple gown. Neither was she wearing a corset under it. She had a stole round her neck which reminded me of Miss Lilian's cat, and her sagging stomach quite spoilt the line of her dress. She had finally been talked out of wearing the tiara but the high pearl choker that looked as if it was steadily choking her was as grand as any tiara. Her slashed-up shoes could only be seen when she hitched up her skirts to stop her heels from getting caught in the hem, or when she was stepping over a puddle. Mrs Beauchamp looked charming in the oyster satin and the two friends made a splendid exit from the verandah.

I was proud of them all. Perhaps none of them would have won a glamorous granny competition, but they could have been in the line-up at the start, even if some of them weren't grannies.

After we had taken our places at the two long tables that were decorated with Christmassy things, though it was nearly Easter, and had thanked the Lord for what we were about to receive, the waitresses brought each of us a small glass of sherry and inquired whether we wanted soup or a prawn cocktail. Miss May looked startled and asked Mrs James in a loud voice whether it was some sort of fishy drink. Since nobody seemed to know much about prawn cocktails everybody said they would prefer the soup. I hesitated. I had never tried a prawn cocktail but I could have soup any day at home. I felt that the occasion called for something a little more adventurous.

I was still dithering when a message was passed up the table that Mrs Turgoose would like a word and it was urgent. She was way down at the bottom end of the other table.

'What do you want?' I asked, a little abruptly. I was afraid that the girl who was waiting to be told which of the starters I wanted wouldn't be too pleased at being kept hanging about even longer for a decision.

'I've left me bottom teeth behind,' said Mrs Turgoose, drawing down her lower lip and baring a toothless gum.

'But you never wear them,' I reminded her. 'They're in the top drawer of your dresser with all the other bottom teeth you've never worn.' By then everybody was letting their soup get cold while they craned their necks and pricked up their ears to discover what was going on. Several of the girls who were standing at the serving hatch were also wondering what was going on. From the look on their faces I could tell that whatever it was they were firmly on the side of Mrs Turgoose.

'Whether I wear them or not isn't the point,' said Mrs Turgoose querulously. 'The point is I don't like people to think I haven't got any, especially at a do like this.' She flashed a dear-old-lady smile at the waitresses who were closing in to see fair play.

'Do I really have to go back and get them for you?' I pleaded. 'You'll only keep them in their box if I bring them, so I can't really see what good it would do you.' I had, by now, abandoned all hope of a prawn cocktail. Mrs Turgoose flashed another smile at the waitresses, who gripped the soup plates they were carrying, and looked as if they would have liked to tip them over my head.

'Well, all right,' she said in martyred tones. 'But on your own head be it if I'm sick in the night through not digesting me food properly and have to ring for you.' I went back to my place at the table and spooned up the lukewarm soup. I daren't leave it after it had been brought specially for me.

The rest of the evening was without incident. Miss Coombe got into a fluster over helping herself to the brussels and looked as if she wished she'd stayed at home, and Miss May came over queer after she had eaten her turkey, but recovered in time for the pudding. Mrs Marsh asked if there was a drop of Guinness anywhere and on being told that there wasn't she told the waitress in a loud voice what she could do with the glass of wine. But luckily the waitress had a granny of her own and didn't take offence.

Mrs Turgoose waited for the plates to be collected then she stood up and asked whether anybody felt like a bit of a sing-song. Nobody did. She half-heartedly struck up 'For He's a Jolly Good Fellow' but when nobody joined in she quavered to a stop and sat down looking very embarrassed. She sulked quite noticeably for a few minutes after.

Mrs Beauchamp rose to her feet, raised her empty glass and would have made a speech if Mrs Marsh hadn't told her to sit down and shut up for Gawd's sake. She also sulked noticeably for a few minutes.

When the last coffee cup had been cleared (nobody made tea for those who didn't drink coffee) and due thanks had been given to all – including the Lord – who had made the evening such a success, each of the ladies was given a real mink flower in a cellophane box. I didn't get one. The waitress who was distributing them at my end of the table said rather haughtily that there were no more left. I wondered if she was paying me out for not fetching Mrs Turgoose's teeth.

'Well, did you enjoy it?' I asked Mrs Peters, after I had helped her out of the minibus and seen her safely to her door.

'It wasn't bad,' she said grudgingly. 'But I thought some of them waitresses were a stuck up lot, and the savoury balls could have done with being a bit more savoury.' I said goodnight to her, then went along the verandah to make sure that everybody else was all right, and that Joey had come to no harm through being left on his own for an hour or two. And then I went to bed. It had been a long and tiring day.

Part Four

Part Four

Chapter Fifteen

IT WASN'T UNTIL the last of the blue rinse had been finally washed out of Mrs James's hair, and it looked less like wire wool, that I was to discover how lonely she was. That I hadn't known about it before wasn't because of any neglect on my part. She was a woman who didn't make a habit of pouring out her troubles over a cup of tea. Neither was she ever to be found standing with a little group on the verandah eagerly discussing the titbit of the day. None of the residents had known her before she moved in, and even Mrs Turgoose, who prided herself on being a mine of information about other people's affairs, had to admit that Mrs James's past history was a closed book to her, which niggled her very much. She kept herself to herself as much as Miss Coombe did, and didn't even have a budgerigar to talk to.

I knew from the records that she was childless, and that she had been a widow since a year or two before she moved in, but I still had no idea of the loneliness that made her do odd little things when she thought nobody was looking.

It was only after she had a similar virus to the one which Mrs Beauchamp had that I got to know her a great deal better.

I gave her nourishing little meals, hot drinks, cold drinks, and all the things that the doctor ordered, and was very glad when he said that she was well enough to get up, and all she needed to bring the colour back into her cheeks was a trip to the Canary Islands, or a world cruise on the *QE2*. He was only joking, of course. He knew that either was as far from her reach as a journey to the moon.

Her doctor was Irish. He was as squarely built, and as solid, as Miss Harrison's piano, which was now in Stew's workshop, waiting for some stalwart soul to come and carry it away. Stew used to play 'Chinese Chopsticks' on it, and 'Three Blind Mice', but however much he tried to master any of the Beatle numbers it still sounded like 'Chinese Chopsticks' or 'Three Blind Mice'.

Whenever Mrs James's Irish doctor came to see her, or any other of his patients, he brought his car to a screaming halt, scattering the pigeons, and making everybody rush to their windows expecting the worst.

After he had waved to them all he hurled himself into the flat he was visiting, sending knick-knacks flying and slip mats skidding. Then he threw himself onto his patient's bed, almost breaking it in half with his weight, and said things which would have made Hippocrates shake his head sorrowfully, but which bucked the patient up at once. He was the same in his surgery.

'And what's wrong with you that a couple of amputations and a bit of clever brain surgery couldn't cure?' he bellowed at the woman who had come for something to stop her sneezing when the pollen count was high.

'It'll be the bonehouse for you if you go on like this,' he bawled at the man whose waterworks were giving him trouble, but not as much trouble as he imagined they were. His patients left the surgery secure in the knowledge that if they did end up having brain surgery for their hay fever or their waterworks landed them in the bonehouse they were in good hands, and couldn't have chosen a finer doctor to warn them of their fate.

Mothers spoke his name with awe when they were telling other mothers of the miracles he'd worked on their sick children, grannies and grandpas swore that they owed their longevity to the way he'd looked after them, and mums and dads said that he was the best doctor anybody could have, despite the terrible things he said to them when he should have been patting their hand and consoling them. But when the time came that they needed consoling he was there at once, saying just the right words.

Nobody believed him when he told them that he would drop dead one of these days unless a law was passed saying that doctors, like parsons, should only work one day a week. The day he died with awful suddenness the whole town mourned. Even those who were not his patients missed him. He did a great many things for people, as well as doctoring them.

The first I knew about Mrs James's loneliness was when she brushed against her telephone on her way to the kitchen to make a cup of tea. We had drunk quite a lot of tea together during the nights she couldn't sleep because of her virus, and we had talked about a lot of things, but never about her loneliness. It was only when she was well again, and started asking me in when I did the round, and made me a cup of tea if I had time to stay, that I noticed her brushing against her telephone.

It was Mrs Beauchamp's son who had started the trend of telephones around the Lodge. Until then the residents had relied on me to transmit any messages they wanted sent in a hurry. Nobody had thought of having one themselves until Mrs Beauchamp got hers.

When the post office people arrived to do the installation, little groups gathered on the verandah and talked about it. They reminded me of the little groups that had gathered in the terrace where I had lived a long time ago, when one of the neighbours caused a sensation by being the first to have a television. The comments about the television had been as caustic as the comments about the telephone.

'There's some round here as are getting a bit too big for their boots,' said Mrs Turgoose when I went to see her the day after the first telephone was put in. 'The way I see it is, if they can afford one of them things they can afford to buy a house, instead of living here, taking up a flat that somebody else on the list is waiting for.' I said that I didn't think that the cost of having a telephone was anything like the cost of buying a house, and anyway it was Mrs Beauchamp's son who was paying for it to be put in, so that he could ring his mother every morning to see how she was.

'Lucky for some,' sneered Mrs Turgoose. 'It's not everybody that's got a son with money to burn. Pity he can't find something better to do with it than splashing it out on telephones. Easy come, easy go as they say.' Mrs Turgoose hadn't got a son. She hadn't any children at all. And neither did she ever have a telephone.

Mrs Peters was another who had some cutting things to say about people who thought they were better than other people because they'd got a telephone. She gave her family no peace until they clubbed together to get one put in for her and soon there were so many residents wanting telephones that the yellow post office van was a common sight on the forecourt.

Mrs James hadn't had to have hers put in. She inherited it from the previous tenant who only used it once, and that was to tell her daughter that she wasn't feeling well. When the daughter hurried over to find out what was wrong, she was too late. It was left to me to break the news.

'Why don't you move the telephone onto the dresser where you can't brush against it whenever you walk across the room?' I said to Mrs James, when I had seen her doing it a few times. She looked at me for a moment then she started to cry. Though I didn't think I had said anything to make her cry I got a tissue from the box on her bedside table and said I was sorry if I had upset her.

'It isn't you,' she sniffed into the tissue.

'Then what is it?' I asked.

'It's that thing,' she said, glaring at the telephone. 'It

gets on my nerves.' I looked at the telephone. It was a plain old-fashioned black one and as far as I could see there was nothing about it that could either make her cry or get on her nerves. Then I remembered a friend once telling me that she wouldn't have a telephone because she thought that they were a gross intrusion on privacy. When I asked her what she meant she said that she wouldn't dream of asking anybody, except a very good friend, into the house if she was in the middle of a meal, or having a bath, or entertaining her lover, but anybody could invade her home simply by dialling a number.

'Do you get a lot of telephone calls?' I asked Mrs James.

'That's the trouble,' she sniffed. 'I don't get any. It's never rung since I've lived here. It gets on my nerves just sitting there and never ringing.'

'But I still don't understand why you keep brushing against it,' I said. Mrs James gave me a watery little smile.

'It's just a habit I've got into,' she said. 'I got so upset when nobody rang me up that I started knocking against it just to hear it tinkle. I could almost make myself believe that it was going to ring. I know it sounds silly, but you tend to do silly things when you're lonely.' She blew her nose and laughed, but I wasn't laughing. I almost needed a tissue myself.

'But surely you're not as lonely as that,' I said. 'You go out, and you have visitors sometimes.' Not often I knew, but neither did Miss Coombe, and she didn't brush against her telephone every time she went near it. She had had hers put in so that she could ring for the vet if Joey was a bit off colour, or needed his claws trimmed, or his beak shortened.

'That's got nothing to do with it,' said Mrs James, showing signs of bursting into tears again. 'Going out and having visitors doesn't stop you from feeling lonely. It's having nothing left belonging to you that makes you feel lonely. I don't feel that I've got anything to call my own these days. It started after my husband died but it's been getting worse lately. I'm lost to death with having nothing to call my own.' I thought again of Miss Coombe. She was so busy teaching her budgie to talk, and clapping her hands every time a goal was scored that she didn't have time to feel lonely. Even the misery she went through after Billy got eaten by the ginger cat, and when the one before him flew out of the window, was probably better than having nothing to think about at all.

'Why don't you have a budgerigar?' I asked Mrs James. She shook her head.

'We had one once and I just started getting fond of it when it fell off its perch and died. We had a dog as well. My husband thought the world of her. She went off once and didn't come back for a week. My man wouldn't eat and wouldn't go to bed at night. If he heard a dog barking in the distance he would trail for miles to find out if it was her. The day she came home as if nothing had happened I swear that I'd have put a bullet through her if I'd had a gun. My husband wasn't the same after that. The doctors said it was a growth but I still say he'd have been here today if it hadn't been for the dog going off the way she did. I had her put down when he died. I couldn't bear to see her around the place after all the trouble she'd caused.' Her eyes were full of hatred for the dog.

'You must have been very lonely after your husband died,' I said.

'Well, I was, but we had quite a big garden and I looked after that until it got too much for me, then of course I had to give up the house and come and live here. I miss the garden. I like putting things in and watching them grow. It isn't the same in a place like this where you can only look at things that other people have grown.' She was still sniffing when I left her, but she was at least dry-eyed.

The old gardener was still with us. His feet had got so bad over the years that he rode a bicycle, or pushed it, wherever he went. He said he felt safer on it than on his poor old feet. But the gardens were as neat as they had ever been. The roses were pruned, the lawns mown and everything done in its due season. Sometimes at committee meetings it was suggested that he would have to go, but excuses were always made to keep him on. Nobody had the courage to give him notice.

He had stayed single all his life. No woman could have matched the matchless beauty of his beloved Ena Harkness, or been as clinging as the Nellie Moser that wound itself round the arches separating the lawns from the rose gardens. Even if a girl had managed to compete with the velvety Elizabeth of Glamis she would have had to move the marriage bed into the greenhouse before she got him into it. And even then there would have been competition from a languishing lily.

He was on his knees doing something to a row of tender young shoots when I went to tell him about Mrs James. He listened carefully, cupping a hand over a deaf ear, and when I had finished he struggled to his feet. He wiped his hands down his trousers and led me past the shed where he kept his forks and spades and all the other tools he cared for as lovingly as he cared for his gardens. We stopped at a patch of ground outside Mrs James's back door. It wasn't a very big patch, but big enough for her to plant a few things and watch them grow. He told her that it could be made to look very nice in the summer with a bed of pansies and an edging of lobelia and aubretia, and in the autumn there could be a chrysanthemum or two, with a few crocuses in the spring. Even the winter was planned for.

On the dark days of December, and when the new year was cold and miserable, Mrs James sat looking through the catalogues she had written off for from the seed merchants. She never sent off for the seeds. She bought them from Woolworth's whenever she had a shilling or two to spare. She read the seed catalogues as I read the travel brochures I sent off for after Christmas. Not with any hopes of realizing the impossible dreams they conjured up but because they made good escapist reading.

She never needed to brush against her telephone again. The old gardener saw to that. It was only to be expected that he would drop in occasionally to ask how her garden grew, and to bring little cuttings from his greenhouse. Sometimes he would bike back after he had been home and had his supper, and go through the catalogues with her, advising her on what seeds she should buy if only she had the money to buy them. There were times when he came back before he had his supper and she shared hers with him. He rang her up at weekends to warn her that there was frost in the air, and to tell her what to do to protect her baby buds from getting nipped.

He felt safe with Mrs James. He knew she wouldn't be expecting him to marry her just because he dropped in to see her now and then. And I was grateful to him. I didn't like the residents bursting into tears when I did the rounds. It was as bad for me as it was for them.

Chapter Sixteen

Long, long ago, when I was doing my training, a sister for whom we had the greatest respect, and who must obviously have been born before her time, told her nurses that she didn't believe in making too many rules. She said that since rules were only for breaking she thought the less there were the happier everybody would be. Consequently she allowed her nurses to eat behind the kitchen door so long as she didn't catch them at it, and she let the patients' visitors sit on the beds on condition that they jumped up the moment they saw her coming, and meticulously straightened the ruffled counterpane. She turned a deaf ear when the domestics ran to her with true stories of the dreadful things the nurses did when her back was turned, and nobody was sent to the matron for talking to the patients, except if the talking interfered with the ward work.

The charitable body had much the same attitude to

rules. Except for the one forbidding four-legged friends to darken the doors, and the other which stressed that even a female visitor shouldn't share a bed for longer than a week, or a fortnight at most, there was nothing the residents were not allowed to do that they might suddenly have been seized with the urge to do. The condition that applicants for a flat should be sober, clean and of good order still obtained, but since all that was gone into before they took up residence, the risk of the peace being disturbed, or necks staying unwashed, was considerably reduced. No limits were set on the time the residents came in at night, and so long as gentleman friends were seen off the premises on the day they arrived, there were no restrictions put on their visits. Hence nobody was ever caught flagrantly violating the rules.

Nevertheless, and in spite of there being no actual laws against them, there were one or two things that went on which the charitable body might not have approved of if they had been aware they were happening. I thought it wiser never to mention in the monthly reports that the moment the off-licence over the bridge threw open its doors I clanked across with a bag of empties and came back with fresh supplies. Miss May craved for a drop of milk stout when she came over queer, and as she came over queer every day, usually just when the off-licence was due to open, it was the least I could do to satisfy the craving. Old Mrs Hunt, who lived in the corner opposite Miss Coombe, liked a daily ration of brown ale, which kept her pecker up, she said. It eased my work considerably if peckers were kept up, so I willingly went across to the off-licence when Mrs Hunt showed signs of drooping.

Neither did I mention at the meetings about Mrs Marsh and Mrs Beauchamp going off to bingo every Wednesday. I felt that, like Miss Coombe, the charitable body might have taken an uncharitable view of it. Miss Coombe had scruples about such things. It was debatable whether she, or the committee either for that matter, would have approved of Mrs Marsh shuffling to my back door once or twice a week with a bribe in one hand and a folded slip of paper in the other. The bribe was usually a small bunch of flowers she had managed to pick when the gardener wasn't looking. The folded slip of paper had the name of the favourite for one of the day's big races scrawled across it.

'Be a sport, mate, and give my Bill a ring and ask him to put a bob each way on this,' she would say, handing me the bribe and the betting slip. Her Bill worked in one of the betting shops in the town.

The pricking of my conscience told me that I should have refused the bribe and returned the slip, but I never did. I accepted both, and even invited Mrs Marsh in and sat her in my mother's old chair while I phoned her Bill. He was always very touched that I should take the trouble to be bookie's runner for his mother's bets. In token of his gratitude he sometimes invited me to have a bob each way myself, but I never did. I felt that it would be a bad example for a matron to set.

But once a year I threw discretion to the winds and encouraged a spate of gambling that caused excitement to run at fever pitch. On the eve of the Grand National I carefully wrote down the names of the runners on small scraps of paper and threw the scraps into a pudding basin which I took with me on the first round the following day. All those who didn't have scruples were invited to dip into the basin and draw out one of the scraps. In return for each dip they had they gave me sixpence. The annual event created certain difficulties.

Respecting Miss Coombe's scruples I never offered her the basin but left it outside her door while I went in to inquire how she was. Though there was no fear of me leading her into temptation, I was afraid she might have looked so shocked at the thought of such depravity that

I would have to abandon the sweepstake, which would have disappointed those who enjoyed a little flutter once a year. Neither did I confront Mrs James with the basin. She also had scruples.

It always took Mrs Peters a long time to make her selection from the scraps that were left when I got round to her. She fumbled around, unfolded three or four and read them. If none of the names coincided with the tips that were given in her newspaper that morning she put them back and brought out a fresh lot. Only after she had drawn a horse that stood a reasonable chance of finishing the course would she hand over her sixpence.

Miss Macintosh, with her good Scottish sense of value, invariably asked whether she could have two dips for ninepence, and Mrs Marsh and Mrs Beauchamp would have snapped up every scrap of paper that was left if they'd had enough sixpences to pay for them.

Miss May dipped her delicate fingers into the basin, saying how wicked she felt at doing anything so daring, then asked me whether I would very much mind making her a cup of something hot to replace the energy she'd used up while she was dipping.

When the race was due to start an unusual hush came over the Lodge. There were no comings and goings along the verandah, except by those who had scruples. Heavy curtains were drawn across windows so that the afternoon light wouldn't spoil the picture on television, and those without a television set sat by their wirelesses groaning when their horse got over one of the fences before its rider, and jumping up and down with excitement if it was still there at the last bend.

I also drew my curtains and watched the race, and when the results were officially shown, and while the sweating victors were being cosseted with blankets and cuddled by their ecstatic owners, who were better off by several thousand pounds, I went across and shared out the winnings. The first prize was never more than five shillings, or twenty-five pence in the new money, but whoever won it was envied and talked about for the rest of Grand National day. Knowing this I always made sure that I never picked a winner myself. I fixed the race so that the horse I had drawn either came in last or not at all.

The year that Mrs Turgoose had two dips from the basin and came up with the first and second winner feelings ran high round the Lodge. There was talk of collusion between the organizer of the draw, which was me, and the winner of thirty-seven and a half pea, which was Mrs Turgoose. I was hurt by the totally unfounded accusations but Mrs Turgoose rose above them. She ignored the rumours that were flying around and bustled into the town, spreading the news of her good fortune wherever she went. The fortune grew larger by the minute.

When one of the junior reporters on the local paper heard from his granny that a lady who lived at the Lodge had won thousands in the Irish sweepstake, he saw it as a way of becoming editor-in-chief in one fell scoop. He dashed round without prior notice to the address his granny had given him and fell panting through Mrs Turgoose's door. I didn't know he was there until Stew came and told me. He said that though I was the boss and he was only the handyman he thought it was my duty to be present at the interview to ensure that nothing was offered for publication that would antagonize the committee or cause ill-feeling among the other residents. Stew knew as well as I did that Mrs Turgoose could be very indiscreet at times. I thanked him for warning me and got across as fast as I could.

Mrs Turgoose wasn't pleased to see me. She knew that I was only there to cramp her style. She had already made the reporter a cup of tea and was embarking on a long rigmarole about the powers of extra-sensory perception that had led her to picking not one, but two winning scraps of paper out of the basin on Grand National day. The young man looked very perplexed until I explained that she had won thirty-seven and a half pea on our own little draw and not thousands of pounds in the Irish sweepstake. All his dreams of becoming editor-in-chief faded, but instead of putting his notebook and pencil away and returning to base to confess that his granny had misled him, he decided to cut his losses and make the best of a bad job. He had the brilliant idea of writing a short cameo on Mrs Turgoose's long life. She gave him enough to write a book and needed no urging to follow chapter by chapter. I sat and listened as the story unfolded. It wasn't washday and the plastic flowers were sparkling clean and tastefully arranged in their plastic containers. The reporter was flanked by a room-high, rubbery-looking rubber plant and an aspidistra, both growing in artificial soil.

'You're a widow I believe,' said the young man in a suitably dismal voice.

'I am,' said Mrs Turgoose, and was off. She recalled the days when her late husband had plodded more than twenty miles to work every morning with hardly any shoes on his feet, and had plodded home again when his day's work was done. The young reporter managed to keep a stiff upper lip, and so did I. I knew for a fact that Mrs Turgoose's very late husband – he had been dead for nigh on forty years – was a milkman almost to the day he died. The only walking he ever did was the short distance from his horse's head to the back of the milk float where he ladled out his customers' pintas from a very large churn. Mrs Turgoose had once laughingly told me that he had never needed to goad the horse to action. They had done the milk round together for so long that the poor old nag could have done it alone, and with both eyes shut, even stopping at the public house where they regularly took their refreshment.

'Of course, that was in the days when the town was overrun with highwaymen, and Russians with their dancing bears.' I listened in amazement. It was the first I'd heard of either highwaymen or Russians with dancing bears. But Mrs Turgoose was in full flood. The Russians, she said, lived only a stone's throw from where we were sitting at that very moment. It was a common sight to see them queuing at the corner shop for honey to give to the bears. It was an even more common sight, she hinted, to see the lusty young Russians, presumably without their bears, chasing after the local girls. From the leering wink she gave him, the embarrassed young man was left in no doubt that the lady he was interviewing had not only been chased by many a Russian but had been caught more than once.

Steadfastly avoiding my eye, Mrs Turgoose went on to tell highly imaginative stories of highwaymen who robbed the rich, and the poor as well, while they were crossing the town moor on their horses. Again she hinted that she had had more than her purse pinched when she was taking an innocent walk across the moor.

It was only after she had run out of the more sensational happenings in her life that Mrs Turgoose started relating things that I knew to be true. She told sad stories of the days when people were so poor that they often didn't have enough to eat, when poverty meant more than having to go without a new mangle when the old one was dropping to pieces and envying the neighbours their annual week's holiday when even a day out was beyond your pocket.

She recalled the days when officials came from the board of guardians, and if they thought there were too many children for the mother to cope with and feed properly they whisked the youngest ones off to the workhouse.

'When that happened,' she said, 'their mothers used to borrow a few shillings, or pawn something and take the baby to Great Ormond Street Children's Hospital.'

'But why did they take the baby there?' asked the reporter, turning over another page.

'Because once they got it there it couldn't be sent to the workhouse,' said Mrs Turgoose.

'And what happened to it then?' asked the young man, beginning to see himself as a sub-editor at least, on the strength of the human story he would be taking back to the office.

'They kept it there,' said Mrs Turgoose. He still wasn't satisfied.

'But how could they keep it there if there was nothing wrong with it?' he asked.

'But there always was something wrong with it,' replied Mrs Turgoose. 'You could bet your life in them days that if the family was poor enough to have to pawn something to get a shilling or two to pay the fare to London, the new baby, and perhaps a few of the other kids as well, would have things wrong with them which they either died of or would never get over properly.'

However sceptical I might have been about highwaymen on the moor, and Russians rushing to the corner shop for honey to give their dancing bears, I knew that the story of mothers taking their babies to Great Ormond Street was true. I had heard similar stories from the older residents who had themselves bundled their children into a train and taken them out of reach of the men from the board of guardians. One of the stories was told me by Mrs Hunt, who lived in the corner opposite Miss Coombe.

Mrs Hunt was ninety. She had a deaf and dumb son. She told me that when he got ill while he was still a very small baby she had dreaded that he might have been taken to the workhouse. She had pawned her husband's best pair of boots and bought a ticket to King's Cross station. She had wrapped the baby in anything warm she could find round the house and dodged the officials who were already on their way to weed out the weakly ones in the family.

Outside the station there was a small group of old men with handcarts, rackety prams and pushchairs who for a penny would push the sick little baby along the road and to the hospital that boasted it never turned a child away. The old men were the equivalent of cabbies, except that their fares were more down to earth, and they reserved the right to keep their vehicles for the use of children only.

When the baby was warmly tucked in his cot the ward sister told Mrs Hunt she could go home, and promised to keep her informed of her son's progress. The sister knew from experience that there was little likelihood of the baby being visited while he was in her care. Better uses could be found for money got from pawning boots than squandering it on visits to a baby who might never go home again.

Once a week the postman delivered a card to Mrs Hunt with a short medical bulletin couched in simple terms, and spaces left to record anything outstanding that might have happened to the baby since the last bulletin was sent. None of the cards mentioned that the little boy would be deaf and dumb.

When a card was delivered saying that Mrs Hunt could fetch her baby home she pawned something else and went off to fetch him. The sister who explained about the complications that had set in after the original illness was cured had sat her on a chair and given her a nice cup of tea to help her get over the shock. But Mrs Hunt told me that she remembered crying all the way home in the train.

The son grew to be a fine fellow. He came to the Lodge every week to see his mother, and except for being deaf and having to talk with his hands he was no different from any of the other sons who came to see her. It was just a pity that he had to have meningitis when there were no antibiotics to stop things getting out of control. Mrs Hunt said that he'd been quite a handful to rear. It was a lot harder for children like him in the days before specialists put their mind to thinking up ways of helping the deaf to hear and the dumb to be more articulate.

I had been told another story of a child so severely

handicapped that he was kept hidden for years so that the authorities wouldn't take him away. But that was too sad even for me to think about.

After Mrs Turgoose had finished enthralling the reporter with stories from her past, true or false, he put his notebook and pencil away and said he would send round a photographer to take a picture of her, just in case he got his article in the next issue. Mrs Turgoose gave him a leering wink and said that a nice young man like him shouldn't have any trouble getting his article in, and he went on his way, ruefully rubbing the spot where she had dug him with her elbow.

The result of the lengthy interview was an eighth of a column slightly overshadowed by an account of a particularly thrilling encounter between two drunks on the previous Saturday night. It skimmed lightly over the Russians and their dancing bears, dwelt briefly on the good old days but concentrated mainly on the brisk way in which the matron had reminded Mrs Turgoose of something she'd forgotten to mention. The word 'brisk' was ill-chosen. It gave those who didn't know me the same impression that the waitresses at the belated Christmas dinner had formed. The paper had a wide circulation, and such was the power of the press that I was looked at coldly for a long time afterwards by readers who believed that I went around being brisk with old ladies, whereas in fact I was really quite timid, especially with Mrs Peters, who terrified me.

Chapter Seventeen

IN SPITE OF Mrs Turgoose's continuing role as matron's nark, her readiness to fill me in with the lesser-known details of an incoming resident's past and her wildly inaccurate guesses at who would be next on the list for admission, she wasn't the woman she had been when I first went to work at the Lodge. A short sharp illness had slowed her down. She spent more of her time sitting by the fire and concocting scandals than she spent going out and unearthing them at their source. She relied more and more on friends popping in to tell her who had been seen cheating at dominoes, being huffed at draughts and concealing a spade up their sleeves when spades were being trumped.

But though the short, sharp illness had robbed her of some of her strength, it hadn't blunted her wit, or made her brain less agile. When her doctor suggested that a week or two at a convalescent home was just what she needed to put her back on her feet, she at once got in touch with a member of the church she only went to when names were being taken for harvest festival hampers. Wires were pulled, and wheels set in motion until a place was found for her in a select little convalescent home at a seaside resort that had once been the playground of princes.

The home was described in the brochure as eminently suitable for invalid gentlewomen of reduced circumstances. It was run by a different charitable body from the one that ran the Lodge, and had special provisions for those who couldn't afford to pay. Mrs Turgoose couldn't afford to pay, and she would have been the last to call herself a gentlewoman, but she packed two sets of clean underwear, a frilly nightdress and a matching frilly bedjacket, and went off to the home for invalid gentlewomen. I used my day off the first week she was there to go and visit her.

When I arrived at the home, which was a long way from the station, Mrs Turgoose was sitting in an elegantly appointed room, hedged in on all sides by invalid gentlewomen. Despite the new dressing gown and the new pair of fluffy slippers she was wearing, there was something about her that set her apart from the others.

'Stuck up lot they are in here,' she said, dunking a ginger biscuit into the rather pallid cup of tea she was drinking. I noticed that the little finger of the hand she held the cup in was crooked almost to breaking point. This was something she must have picked up from the gentlewomen. I had never seen her do it before. I also noticed that she was wearing her bottom teeth, which I gathered was why she was dunking the biscuit. Biting into a hard ginger biscuit required the full cooperation of upper and lower teeth. Mrs Turgoose had never been able to manage her bottom dentures. She leaned forward in her chair.

'See that old girl sitting in the corner?' she said, indicating with her thumb an elegantly dressed lady who looked every inch a gentlewoman.

'Yes, but keep your voice down,' I said, 'she can hear every word you say.'

'I think she's a bit funny in the head,' said Mrs Turgoose, lowering her voice slightly. 'She sits there all the time reading one of them posh papers and doing crosswords. The only time she moves is to go to the you-know-where, and when I walk over to have a word with her. When she sees me coming she gets up quick and goes over to the chair in the other corner. They all do that. I'm beginning to think it's a place for that sort of thing instead of a proper convalescent home like they said it was going to be.'

A tall woman wearing a kimono, and smoking a

cigarette through a slim holder, came towards us while Mrs Turgoose was whispering. She quickened her step and turned her head as she passed.

'See what I mean?' said Mrs Turgoose. 'She's hardly looked my way since I've been here. And she's always smoking them funny cigarettes. From the smell of them I wouldn't be a bit surprised if it was drugs she was in here for.' Marijuana was already making big news in the Sunday papers, and though Mrs Turgoose couldn't pronounce the word she knew that smoking it was only one step away from utter ruin. I said that I thought it was highly unlikely that the home for invalid gentlewomen would be part of the drug scene: and even she admitted that you wouldn't expect to come across hippies in a place like that.

'But whether it's drugs or not it doesn't stop her from being civil. She's no right to look straight through me as if I wasn't here.' After one or two gentlewomen had walked past with their heads averted I began to wonder whether they were indeed wishing that Mrs Turgoose wasn't there. Having to convalesce with somebody who nudged and winked and fell about laughing at even the most feeble joke could be very trying. The gentlewomen might also have had difficulty in understanding some of the jokes which Mrs Turgoose told them, especially those where the nudges and winks were necessary to emphasize the double meaning.

I didn't go to the home again until the last week of Mrs Turgoose's stay. She had dropped me a very vulgar postcard which Dai the Post read and commented on when he delivered it, saying that she hoped it found me well as it left her at present and would I take her a clean pair of knickers and a bunch of plastic flowers when I went to bring her home. Yours Truly, Polly Turgoose.

She was waiting on the drive when I got there. With her was the lady who had sat so aloofly in the corner on my first visit, and also the one who had swept by smoking the cigarette in the slim holder.

'Here you are at last,' exclaimed Mrs Turgoose in a very ladylike voice. 'We reely began to think you wasn't coming.' I apologized for being there exactly on time. She looked me up and down in a critical way. 'I should have thought you'd have come in a hat and a pair of gloves,' she said uppishly. 'Ladies don't usually go about without hats and gloves.' I noticed that she and the two gentlewomen were wearing hats and gloves. I suddenly felt very conspicuous.

Mrs Turgoose loftily introduced me to her new friends but I didn't quite catch their names. I got the feeling that she wasn't too sure of them herself.

'We are just going into the town for a cup of tea,' she said, smirking warmly at them but not at me. 'Please yourself, but you can come if you like.' I said I'd be delighted to go and followed the three women, shifting the carrier bag containing the knickers and the plastic flowers from one hand to the other when it was in danger of being jostled by somebody hurrying past. We were walking at a very slow pace. Whenever we came to a cross roads or stepped off a pavement I was surprised to see the two gentlewomen tenderly holding on to their fellow-patient as if she was a piece of fragile china. I knew she had been quite ill but that was several weeks ago, and after a period of convalescence and some good sea air, I hadn't expected her still to be in such a weak state that she needed helping off pavements.

At a genteel café in the town we had a pot of tea for four and some buttered scones. The butter was spread very thinly. I would have preferred one of the cream slices, or a piece of the chocolate gateau that the waitress tried to tempt us with, but nobody but me was tempted so I settled for a scone.

Throughout the dainty little meal the two ladies threw compassionate looks at Mrs Turgoose and kept asking her if she was quite sure she was warm enough, and whether the scones were to her liking. She first asked for a window on the far side of the café to be opened, then for it to be shut again. She begged for another small scone, saying that as it might be her last she had better make the most of it. The ladies exchanged pitying glances. I understood Mrs Turgoose to mean that it would be the last scone she would be eating in the café as she was going back to the Lodge later that day, and saw nothing in the remark to arouse pity. As usual I was wrong.

Back in the convalescent home she changed her knickers, then, with great ceremony, she halved the bunch of plastic flowers and divided them between the two ladies who had accompanied us to the café. They seemed quite overcome by the floral tribute. They each dabbed their eyes and kissed Mrs Turgoose warmly, then turned away, too choked with emotion to speak.

'A nice lot of women they were in there,' she said, when we were sitting in the train on our way back to the Lodge. 'Especially the two we went out with this morning.'

'But I thought you said they were a stuck-up lot and a bit funny in the head,' I said crossly. I was still feeling peeved at the way she had greeted me when she saw me without either a hat or gloves, and the way she had ignored me while we were eating the scones.

'Yes, well, they didn't have much to say when I first

got there but they were a lot nicer to me after I told them that I'd got something wrong with me that the doctors couldn't get to the bottom of, and nobody knew how to cure.' I stared at her, aghast.

'But that's not true,' I said. 'All you had was a virus, and you were cured almost at once with the antibiotics I had to give you every four hours – and through the night as well,' I reminded her nastily.

'Well, they weren't to know that, were they?' she said. 'And when I told them that I might only have six months to live, they couldn't do enough for me.' I knew then why Mrs Turgoose had been led so gently to the café, and why her passing allusion to the last scone she would be eating had been taken so seriously, and why the gift of the plastic flowers had been more than the two ladies could bear. I didn't speak for the rest of the journey. I was too shocked.

But Mrs Turgoose had a lot longer than six months to live, though there were those at the Lodge who hadn't. When Mrs Marsh rang her bell one night to tell me that she was going to die and she thought I'd better send for her family, my heart sank, not only because I couldn't imagine the Lodge without Mrs Marsh but because I knew at once that she should go into hospital, and getting her there would be difficult, if not impossible.

Nobody ever wanted to go into hospital. However ill they were, they begged to be allowed to stay in their own bed and die there if the worst came to the worst. When this wasn't possible and the ambulance men struggled with their stretchers through narrow doorways or up difficult stairs, I always felt guilty at letting them take the patient away. But there were limits to what could be done with mostly only me to do it. I propped Mrs Marsh up on her pillows to ease her breathing and promised that I would ring her family and tell them she wasn't well.

'I'm going to send for the doctor first,' I told her. 'I think he'll want you to go into hospital.' She raised herself on one elbow and glared at me.

'I ain't going to no hospital, neither for you nor anybody else, so it's not a bit of use sending for the doctor. I'll stop here where I belong.' She sank back, exhausted with her little outburst.

When the doctor came he held her hand very gently in his and spoke to her in the voice he used when he was talking to nice old ladies who were nearing their end. He didn't know Mrs Marsh as well as I did. She had never been a nice old lady. She was an extremely rough diamond and I was very fond of her.

'I'm going to send you to hospital for a day or two,' he said, thinking in his innocence that she wasn't perfectly aware that she was dying. 'They'll be able to do more for you than we can here.' She snatched her hand out of his and pushed it down the bed where he couldn't get at it.

'You're going to do nothing of the sort,' she said. 'I'm not going to no hospital and that's final. They can do no more for me there than my folks and the matron can do for me here. I shan't keep me finger on the bell like that Miss May does, asking for this and that. And you know as well as I do that I shan't be here much longer to trouble anybody.' The doctor opened his mouth to say more but I gave him a warning look. He wrote out a prescription for things that wouldn't do anything to stop Mrs Marsh dying but would make it easier for her, then he patted the hand that wasn't pushed down the bed, and told her he'd be in to see her in the morning. But she wasn't listening.

'Do you think you can cope if we don't send her to hospital?' he asked anxiously when we were outside. He knew that I shouldn't have to, and I knew that I couldn't, but I knew very well that I would. I tried not to think of the hours I would spend at night when her relations couldn't be there, listening to her trying to breathe, instead of listening to her telling me funny things that had happened to her when she was young. I knew how my back would ache with lifting her up, lying her down, and turning her this way and that to make sure that she was as comfortable as anybody dying could ever be.

'Yes, I'll manage,' I told the doctor. 'She's got relations who will come in when they can and take turns with sitting with her at night. And the district nurse will come in twice a day. We'll manage somehow.'

'It won't be for long,' he said, getting into his car.

His words were intended to give me comfort and assurance. But they gave me neither. I was much too fond of Mrs Marsh to be comforted by the thought that she wouldn't be with us much longer. Her slashed-up shoes and Cockney wit had made her very special. I knew there would never be another like her.

She had been ill for less than a month when her family came to thank me for letting her stay at the Lodge instead of sending her to hospital.

'She'd never slept anywhere but in her own bed except for when the war was on and she had to sleep in the shelters. And she never slept even then,' they told me. 'She'd have died of shock if she'd had to go into hospital.'

Mrs Beauchamp couldn't for the life of her think what had happened to her friend. On the day of the funeral she stood beside me watching the cortege go by. It was bitterly cold and she was wearing her extremely old mink coat and a great deal of jewellery.

'Whatever is it, dear?' she asked, a trifle peevishly. 'And why are we standing about like this in the cold?' She had long ago lost all track of time, and until her friend became too ill to help her, she had relied more and more on Mrs Marsh to keep her abreast with current affairs. Without her there to give her a running commentary she could find no explanation in her muddled mind for the procession that was passing us at a snail's pace.

'It's Mrs Marsh,' I whispered. She peered round at the small crowd that had gathered.

'How can it possibly be Mrs Marsh when she's nowhere to be seen?' she asked, with a touch of imperious irritability in her voice. 'You must go and find her at once, and tell her that she is missing all the excitement of seeing the dear Viceroy driving past.' As well as the time she had spent in the copper belt, Mrs Beauchamp had lived for a year or two in India, and though she had only the vaguest memory of what she had been doing five minutes after she did it, she had the most vivid memories of the days when she had stood waving flags while the Viceroy made triumphant entries and exits. The present scene was stirring those memories.

I did all I could to make her understand that it was Mrs Marsh who was keeping us shivering on the forecourt and not the Viceroy, but she took no notice and insisted on clapping her hands and shouting 'Hurrah' as the hearse went by. She even sang a bar or two of 'God Save the King' until quelled with a nudge from Mrs Turgoose and some dirty looks from all sides. She had forgotten that the King had died more than twenty years ago and it was his daughter she should have been asking God to save.

When the last car and its mourners had disappeared from our sight I took Mrs Beauchamp back to her flat and made some coffee. I wasn't going to the funeral. I was suffering terribly with lumbago, which the doctor said was the result of too much heavy lifting. Mrs Marsh had always been a well-built lady.

Mrs Beauchamp looked everywhere for her friend. She was very cross when she couldn't find her.

'I do wish she wouldn't go off like this without telling anybody,' she said. 'Even if she's gone into the town to get something nice for our tea she could have told me she was going.'

'Perhaps she wasn't sure herself that she was going until the last minute,' I said.

'She shouldn't have gone then, should she?' said Mrs Beauchamp. 'She must have known how worried

I'd be. For all we know she could have broken her leg, or be lying dead somewhere.' I nodded sadly.

Shortly after that we were standing in respectful silence watching Mrs Beauchamp starting on her final journey. She hadn't enjoyed anything very much after her friend went. Her son Evelyn wanted her to go home with him, but she said she would rather stay where she was. She would have hated not to be there when dear Mrs Marsh came back.

The bosom friends were sadly missed.

Chapter Eighteen

I HAD BEEN working at the Lodge rather less than ten years when I had to leave it for a while to have a bit of minor surgery done at the hospital where I was once a staff nurse.

The years had been as all years are: one or two very good or very bad, but most of them so-so. There were setbacks, but none that I didn't worry myself to death over until they came right in their own mysterious ways.

There had been several frights and many small miracles. I never got over the fear of answering an emergency bell, wondering what I should find when I opened the door of whoever had rung for me. On one occasion there hadn't even been an emergency bell. I was sitting one morning having a nice little chat with Mrs Judd when she gave me a peculiar look which didn't warn me that she was about to end the conversation with an abruptness that left me staring down at her in disbelief. Mrs Judd had always boasted that she had never had a day's illness in her life. She would have been glad not to have spoilt her record.

I was always grateful for the miracles. I could never believe my luck when some sort of inner voice told me to go across and see somebody, and I got there just in time to avert disaster, or I got there in time to be able to say I was there when the disaster happened. When the inner voice told me to go and see Mrs Jackman I obeyed without hesitation. Mrs Jackman was in her kitchen. The gas burner she had forgotten to light was full on and there was a strong smell everywhere. It was then that arrangements were made to have safety cookers put in every flatlet. They were often so safe that they wouldn't light at all, but at least nothing dire could happen when an old lady forgot to strike a match.

This was before the days when the Lodge was alive with men changing us to natural gas. 'I don't want to be changed to natural gas,' complained Mrs Peters. 'I'm all right as I am.' Changing her to natural gas took time and patience. The gas men did as her family had so often done: they drew straws to decide which of them should sacrifice themselves for the cause of North Sea gas. The ones upon whom the lot fell walked into her flatlet full of forebodings. They knew they would get several lashes from her tongue before they crept out again.

During the years, I had twice been the bride's mother, and four times the doting grandma who truthfully believed that the newest arrival was the most beautiful baby in the world. I had also been burgled.

Being burgled isn't nice, especially when it happens the night before you have planned to go on holiday. I had got up in the morning full of the joys of going to the Isle of Wight for a fortnight, only to find that a burglar had nipped into the downstairs bathroom window and helped himself to my holiday money, and a lot more besides. I was very upset. I had been looking forward to going to the Isle of Wight for a fortnight. I still went, after the policemen had finished taking fingerprints, but it wasn't the carefree holiday that I had expected it to be. I kept waking in the night wondering why I, who had always been a light sleeper, hadn't heard myself being robbed. When I got home I found myself looking with deepest suspicion at the most unlikely people, wanting to ask them if it was they who had scrambled into the bathroom window and out of the back door, taking with them my hard-earned savings.

When I told the residents about the bit of minor surgery I was going to have, the news was received in various predictable ways. The rounds I did were pepped up by breathless accounts of similar operations to the one I was having, which had gone decidedly wrong. According to most of the accounts my days were numbered, or would be considerably curtailed.

Those who remembered well every detail of an identical surgical experience they had undergone thirty or forty years before gave me harrowing word pictures of the tortures, the hovering for months at death's door and the awful despair when it was discovered that in a momentary lapse the surgeon had removed the wrong bit and it all had to be done again. They were quick to remind me that I wasn't as young as I once was and there were many things that could go wrong while I was innocently sleeping on the operating table. Fortunately I had seen so many things go right in my years as a nurse that I wasn't too bothered by the doom-laden warnings.

As was to be expected, Miss May was greatly saddened by the news. She rained kisses on my hand, dabbed her eyes and begged me to tell her what the chances were of somebody answering her emergency bell when she came over queer in the night and needed a cup of something hot to stay her. I told her that the deputy matron who would be in charge while I was away was a very kind lady who would leap into action the moment she heard a bell, at whatever time of the day or night it was rung. But Miss May still wasn't happy. Would the deputy matron be prepared to go clanking to the off-licence every morning and bring back the milk stout she so desperately craved, and which was vitally necessary to keep body and soul together? I said I was sure she would if she was approached in the proper manner, by which I meant that she would have to be a very strong-minded lady not to be wheedled into doing it as I had been wheedled into doing so many small favours for Miss May. Then Miss May had another terrifying thought. What if I were to die, she said, and never go back to the Lodge again. Who then would fill in the forms when she needed to claim for a new set of teeth, or a new pair of spectacles on the Supplementary Benefits? I told her that all such problems would have to be faced if and when they arose, but I assured her that in the event of my not returning to the Lodge for any reason whatsoever the charitable body would see to it that her forms got filled in properly. Miss May was still looking very worried when I left her.

Miss Coombe told Joey about the operation which the poor dear matron would be having shortly, but he wasn't interested. He was busily stabbing at his mirror, and repeating his name and address in a sepulchral voice. Miss Coombe had spent so long making him repeat after her that he was Joey Coombe and he lived at the Lodge that he was word perfect the day he flew out of the window when her back was turned one morning. The man who coaxed him out of a tree, three miles away as the budgie flies, told me later that he couldn't believe his ears when the little bird opened his tiny beak and gave his name and address in a perfectly intelligible croak. The man said that when he heard the little so-and-so talking like a bloke with a frog in his throat he felt as scared as if it had been one of the birds in the Alfred Hitchcock film. He'd got him back quick, he said, not liking the sound of it at all. There was something not quite right about a budgie being so articulate.

Miss Coombe had wept with joy when Joey came home, and had begged his rescuer to sit down for a moment and have a cup of tea while he watched her little friend play a game of football, but the man had declined the invitation and hurried off, muttering something about witchcraft.

Mrs Peters was very cynical when I told her I would be off for a week or two while I was having an operation. She looked closely into my face then, finding no evidence of anything wrong with me, she entered into a lengthy diatribe about people who used imagined illness as an excuse to idle their time away in hospital. She had known a woman once, she said, who had sent in a note to her employers saying that she wouldn't be in because she had something wrong with her, and it was only the very next day that she was seen in the town doing her shopping. But be sure your sins will find you out, said Mrs Peters, it wasn't long before the woman really did have something wrong with her and she was dead and buried within the month; which just went to show that it didn't do to go round saying you'd got something wrong with you when you hadn't. I left her flat full of doubts about my own alleged complaint.

Miss Macintosh dispelled the doubts. She said that she had suspected for a long time that I hadn't been feeling myself. She wasn't in the least surprised to hear that things had come to a head at last. She advised me to put my house in order before I went into hospital so that if anything untoward should happen those who were left would have nothing to worry about. She said she would be happy to give me the name of the donkey sanctuary that had benefited from her cousin's will in case I was in doubt what to do with my own small fortune. She had a twinkle in her eye while she was saying all this. I promised her that I had put my house in order by getting the washing up to date and running a cleaner over the carpet and a duster over the furniture, and as my post office account hardly reached double figures I wouldn't be needing the name of the donkey sanctuary. She wished me well, and said she would look forward to having a glass of something to celebrate my return, even if it wasn't Christmas, and I continued the round in a more optimistic frame of mind. I was able to force a smile at the worst of the forebodings and even managed to raise a laugh at one of them.

Mrs Turgoose's eyes lit up when I gave her a brief outline of the operation I was having. She told me that she had been reading a lot in the Sunday papers lately about operations which in some mysterious way had changed not only the personality of those who had them, but their sex as well, making them grow beards, or bosoms, and other things which they hadn't had before. I said that I didn't think the operation I was having would make me grow a beard and Mrs Turgoose said she thought it was a great pity. I could have earned a fortune, she said, selling my story to the Sunday papers if I'd come out of the hospital with a bit more than I'd gone in with. She gave me a dig in the ribs to make sure that I would know which bit she meant, then she sorted out a few plastic arum lilies and told me to keep my chin up. She said that unless they carried me out of the hospital feet first I had nothing to worry about. I would come back to the Lodge feeling like a new woman, or – nudge nudge, wink wink – a new man if they got their operations mixed up.

They didn't get their operations mixed up and I wasn't carried out of the hospital feet first, but it was quite a while before I went back to the Lodge feeling like a new woman. The residents who had so gloomily warned me that I would be worse before I was better had been absolutely right. As, with the wisdom of age, they usually were.

About the Author

Brought up in Lincolnshire, Evelyn Prentis left home at eighteen to become a nurse. She later moved to London during the war, where she married and raised her family. Like so many other nurses, she went back to hospital and used any spare time she might have had bringing up her children and running her home. Born in 1915, she sadly died in 2001 at the age of eighty-five.

Evelyn published five books about her life as a nurse, and Ebury Press are reissuing them all. *A Nurse in Time*, *A Nurse in Action*, *A Nurse and Mother* and *Matron at Last* are all now available and *Matron in Charge* will follow shortly.

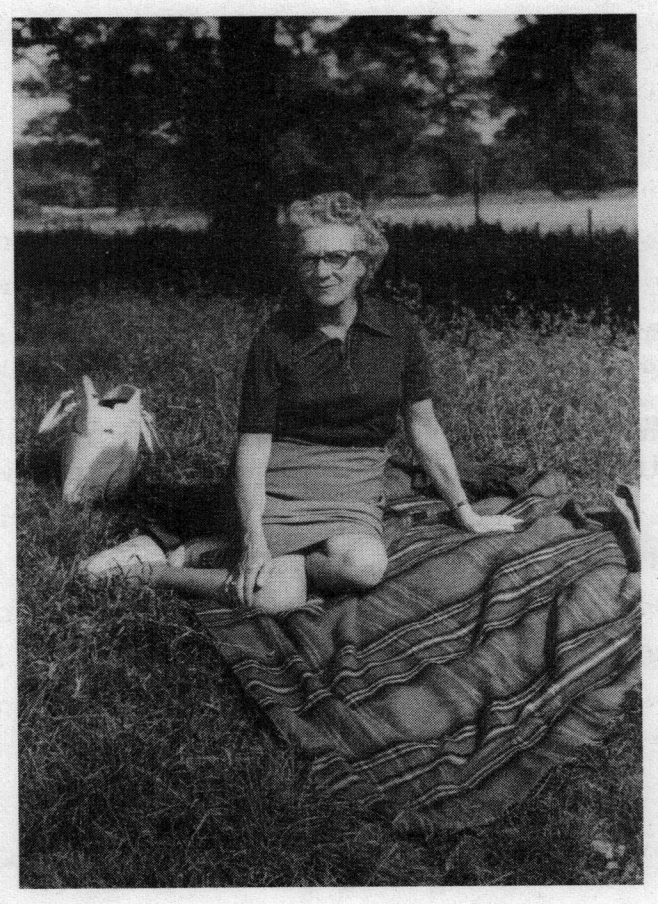

Have you read Evelyn's other books?

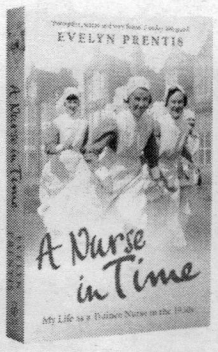

Desperate circumstances were something Evelyn had to get very used to when she began her life as a nurse. In 1934 Evelyn left home for the first time to enrol as a trainee at a busy Nottingham hospital and *A Nurse in Time* is her affectionate and funny account of those days of dedication, hardship and joy.

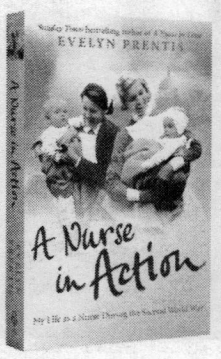

Surprising Matron as well as herself, Evelyn managed to pass her Finals and become a staff-nurse. Encouraged, she took the brave leap of moving from Nottingham to London – brave not least because war was about to break…

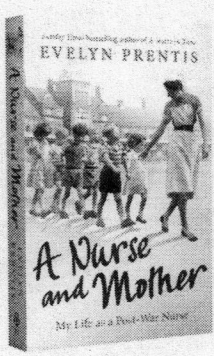

At the end of the Second World War, as husbands came back to Civvy Street their wives had the luxury of staying at home with the children. But soon Evelyn realised she had to find part-time work to make ends meet, and to her astonishment she was offered part-time hours at her old hospital.

And coming soon ...

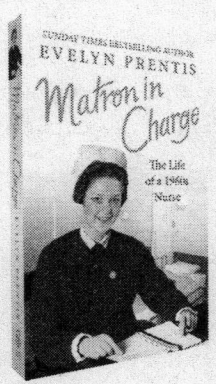

From the door-slamming Miss Cromwell to Mrs Silver's shoplifting and Mrs May coming over all queer, being Matron in charge of the Lodge was rarely straightforward. So when her ladies became unusually united in their grumbling about newest resident Ivy, the woman who'd kept the betting shop on the High Street, Evelyn was ready for all hell to let loose.